The Food and Cooking of China

The Food and Cooking of China

An Exploration of Chinese Cuisine in the Provinces and Cities of China, Hong Kong, and Taiwan

Francine Halvorsen

John Wiley & Sons, Inc.
New York • Chichester • Brisbane • Toronto • Singapore

Library of Congress Cataloging-in-Publication Data:

Halvorsen, Francine.
The food and cooking of China : an exploration of Chinese cuisine in the provinces and cities of China, Hong Kong, and Taiwan / Francine Halvorsen.
p. cm.
Includes index.
ISBN 0-471-11055-8 (paper : alk. paper)
1. Cookery, Chinese. 2. Cookery—China. 3. Cookery—Hong Kong. 4. Cookery—Taiwan. I. Title
TX724.5.C5H343 1996
641.5951—dc20 95-35182

Printed in the United States of America

10 9 8 7 6 5 4 3 2 1

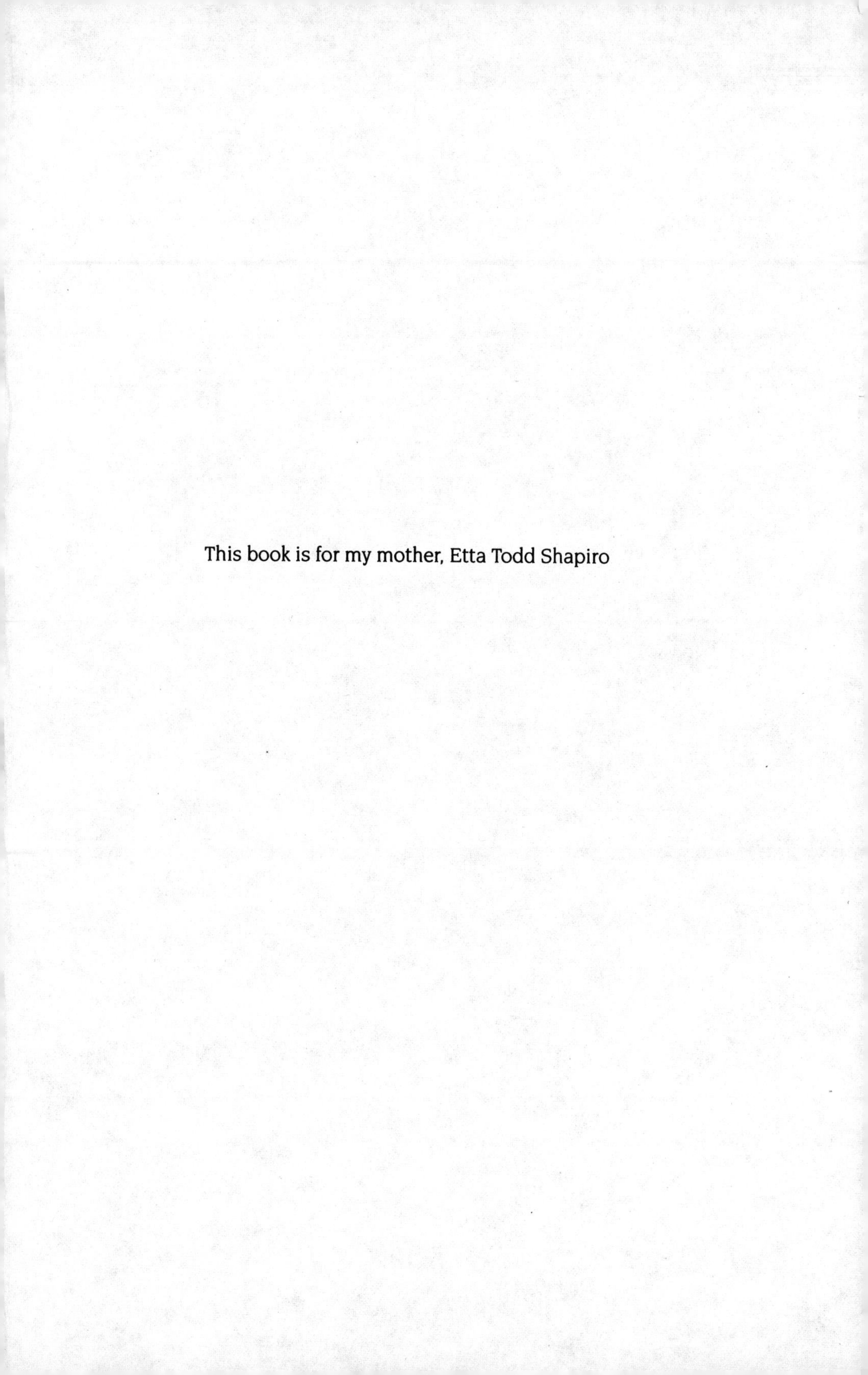

This book is for my mother, Etta Todd Shapiro

ACKNOWLEDGMENTS

This page reflects an embarrassment of riches. No journey, no meal, and no book that emerges from concept to actuality is accomplished alone. Professional colleagues and strangers that were generous were many. *Xie xie nimen*. Thank you all.

In Boston: Lisa Dickason at the ITT Sheraton Corporation understood and expedited itinerary and interview contacts.

In New York: Yung Chun Li and Barbara Wang of China Airlines enhanced a flight that was the best possible. Thanks to: Walt H. Chu of Taiwan Visitor's Association for information and expertise, and Jeanne Dalton of Cathay Pacific and Dragon Air for her enthusiasm and generosity. Grace Swen and her wonderful students at the Chinese Community Center graciously let me share some of their morning language classes.

In Beijing: At the Great Wall Sheraton, Leon Larkin and Yan Zhen Cui facilitated my visit in the midst of a very busy week and saw to it that nothing was overlooked. Eugene Nojek, the American embassy's cultural affairs officer, was kind enough to arrange a banquet of good food and good company. The V.I.P. Bureau Chief, whom I won't embarrass by name, took me for the best lunch ever. And thanks to Zhang Wuwei for his kindness in spending time with a new friend.

In Shanghai: At the Sheraton Hua Ting Hotel, thanks to Joshua Gu, public relations manager, and Tsang Kam Fai, chief of the Chinese kitchen, with whom I would cook and eat and talk any day. Paul Hoeps, former executive chef, directed me to the best chef's store. Dr. Lynne Martin, of the United States Information Service, shared her insights.

In Xi'an: At the Sheraton Xi'an Hotel, I'd like to thank Robert Lee, general manager, James Chow, Mona Guo, and Raj Gupta, the executive chef, who steered me to the best of the old and the new and gave me a glimpse of living history. At the Xi'an Cookery Training Station,

Lin Jianhua, Master, and Liu Jun Ling, Senior Chef, took the time and had the patience to talk to a stranger about T'ang Dynasty cooking and modern eating habits.

In Guilin: At the Sheraton Guilin Hotel, Roger Wright, Lloyd Donaldson, and Sally Yang shared their time, experience, and their good company above and beyond "professional" hospitality. Thanks to Stewart Wee, the executive chef, and Li Siu Chor, the Chinese executive chef, for their patience, knowledge, and skill.

In Hong Kong: I am grateful to Heinz Schmeig, the executive chef of the Sheraton Hong Kong Hotel & Towers, Kowloon, who not only administers to an enormous world-class destination, but has an exemplary style and gives personal attention to detail. Thanks also to Barbara Stiemerling and Paulina De Rosa of ITT Sheraton, Asia, for their time and good will, and to Stephen Wong of the Hong Kong Tourist Association for his wealth of food knowledge.

In Taipei: Jane Lu and Chang Hwa Chou, executive at the Lai Lai Sheraton, are models of excellence and understatement. At the Tourism Bureau, Deputy Director General Hunter H.T. Eu and C.K. Lee, Deputy Director, international division, provided support and knowledge. I am grateful to Felix J. Chen, whose organizational skills I envy and miss, Dr. Clark Hsieh, Chairman of the School of Nutrition, Dr. Kuo-Tung Chen, Professor at the School of Pharmacy at the T'aipei Medical College, and Lily Liang, of the Ritz Hotel, for a memorable dinner. Yang Chi Hua of Din Tai Fung shared an unbeatable evening of art and food. Thanks also to Rita Wong, director of the Foundation of Chinese Dietary Culture, and Teresa Lin, a thoroughly modern food historian and good companion.

Without family and friends, I would never get anything done. To Jesse Halvorsen, Linda Lee, Lionel Halvorsen, and Peggy Hoban, many thanks for the good times cooking, eating, and talking and for your conviction that I could do it. Thanks also for not running from the kitchen and sending out for pizza every time the smoke alarm went off.

Thank you to Juliana Nash for being a good listener at a time when there were far more important things on her plate. A special thank you to Robert Feldman, who encourages my best and even better makes me laugh when it isn't.

At John Wiley & Sons, Claire Thompson is the editor one wishes for and is lucky to get. Maria Colletti and Allison Ort Morvay are the clear, patient voices on the phone who answer sensibly even the silly questions.

Unfortunately the good will of all the above cannot prevent me from making errors, and those are mine.

Francine Halvorsen

Contents

Contents

PREFACE

There are few things more exciting than a journey. The ardent traveler has pleasures at every turn. This book offers an armchair journey with the hope that it will be the impetus for a culinary adventure and maybe a geographical one, as well. As I made my way through various parts of China I was taken by the general responsiveness to my interest in food and by the number of people who welcomed my enthusiasm.

Although there is a high level of connoisseurship among aficionados of Chinese food, the general approach to food is a relaxed appreciation. It is a very forgiving cuisine. The country is large and it has a diverse population living in various environments and they all cook and eat Chinese food. There are over one hundred detailed recipes in this book but you will get an equal amount of information from reading about meals shared and markets visited.

The year is 4693 on the Chinese calendar on my desk. On February 19, 1996 it will be New Year's day, 4694. It seems therefore presumptuous to define dates in the form of "B.C." and "A.D."; instead I use the academically prefered B.C.E. and C.E. referring to common eras as defined in the West.

This book has no map. The truth is that I find it too politically difficult to select one. My education has enabled me to see more than one side at every border but has not prepared me adequately to monitor the disparities drawn by diverse cartographers.

My interest in the food of China stems from my enthusiasm for the poetry and painting of China. Even as a teenager I took courses at the China Institute in addition to ones at the Art Student's League. My degree from Columbia is in Religion with a specialty in East Asian Studies and a lot of take-out food.

To have great chefs you need great eaters. Within reason, I am a fearless taster. I think it is important to mention I was not once upset by any food that I ate on my trip. I also came back wearing the same size six clothes I left with. I ate food that I bought at markets, from street vendors, at 5 A.M. breakfast stalls, and the very finest world class restaurants and never needed any of the stomach remedies friends insisted I take with me. People have asked me how I do it and I tell them the following: 1) I eat only where there are other people eating and smiling; 2) I don't eat anything that looks truly unappealing, unless someone I trust advises it; 3) I travel with alcohol in gel to clean my own hands several times a day; and 4) I trust to a certain amount of instinct and good luck.

In approaching a dish that you haven't tasted before, be brave; after all it is only food. When you shop for Chinese vegetables and products, ask questions. Have fun, take your time—you will still have a meal in pretty short order. Most of the recipes use basic cooking techniques which can be prepared with only a few pots and utensils. This book will help you cook with confidence and pleasure the Chinese food that you thought you couldn't make in your own kitchen. More importantly, I hope you enjoy the journey.

FRANCINE HALVORSEN

INTRODUCTION

Chinese Food *Traditions*

Lao Tzu said, "Handle a large country with as gentle a touch as you would cook a small fish." Tao, or "the way" of Lao Tzu, is a quietism that suggests that "The way to do is to be." It prescribes, "Be careful with speech so as to nourish your virtue. Regulate your food so as to nourish your body."

Throughout Chinese philosophy, few things are more important than speech and food. Mencius (389–305 B.C.E.) said, "Tranquility keeps the words that come out of the mouth from exceeding proper measure, and keeps the food that goes into the mouth from exceeding proper measure. Thus character is cultivated." Scholar gourmets abound.

More than 2,000 years before the remarkable period of the "hundred philosophers" (551–*c.* 233 B.C.E.) that includes Confucius, Lao Tzu, Mencius, and Chuang Tzu, Fu Hsi invented writing. He also invented the nets and baskets needed to maintain the fishing, trapping, and cooking that led to the development of civilization. They are small matters of the largest scope.

Shen Nung, the "divine husbandsman," split a piece of wood for a plowshare and bent a piece of wood for the plow's handle. He domesticated animals, used draft animals to pull the plows, and advanced agriculture. The wooden mortar and pestle, really an early form of the mill, resulted in the change from using whole grain to grinding it into flour for baking. Shen Nung arranged for people from all parts of China to come together in one place with their products and wares and exchange them according to their needs, so that commerce was developed.

The dates of 2852–2737 B.C.E. are traditionally given as the era Fu Hsi and Shen Nung, two legendary cultural heroes of early Chinese history whose importance is still noted today.

Inscriptions on early pots and eating vessels encourage people to nurture the mind and the senses as they eat, and poets observed the potters as they created their vessels.

As a potter may be making clay pots,
  the pieces of clay being quite the same,
Yet there take shape in his hand
  Containers of sugar, milk, clarified butter, and water.

The odes of Confucius mention hundreds of kinds of plants, nut and fruit trees, as well as fish, birds, and animals that serve as a source of provisions.

Fine fish to net,
Ray, skate;
Milord's wine
Is heavy and wet.

Food in plenty,
Say good food;
Plenty of food,
All of it good.

The food itself has symbolic value. The chicken becomes not only a sacred bird used for prophecy and divination, but was called a hero of cuisine by the poet and gastronomic philosopher Yuan Mei (Chi' ing Dynasty). The goose and duck represent fidelity and joy, the pigeon and quail filial devotion, and the fish prosperity, wealth, and regeneration. Oranges and tangerines will keep sweetness in life.

Yuan Mei wrote a book on Chinese cuisine that is still treasured. In it he says:

> Into no department of life should indifference be allowed to creep; into none less than the domain of cookery. Just as a good calligrapher should not overtire his hand nor a poet his brain, so a good cook cannot turn out in one day more than four or five distinct dishes.

He also presses for carefulness and cleanliness.

> Don't cut bamboo shoots with an oniony knife. . . A good cook frequently cleans his knife, frequently changes his cloth, frequently scrapes his board, and frequently washes his hands. If smoke or

> ashes from his pipe, or perspiration from his head, insects from the wall, or dirts from the pan get mixed with the food, though he be a chef among chefs, yet diners would hold their noses and decline.

Chefs and provisioners were given social status and when a new home was built, the kitchen was given the most auspicious position and the rest of the house was built around it. In a continued folk tradition, an image of the Kitchen God, Jo Kwan, hangs over many stoves only to have his lips smeared with honey and burned annually to spread sweet words.

Even simple food has been dignified. The Sung Dynasty poet Mei Yao Che wrote:

> The girl who sells melons beside the stream
> Gathers her melons in the fields on the hillsides.
> She does not need to spin hemp.
> She has handsful of bronze money.

The food and cooking of China is one of the oldest continuous culinary traditions in the world, its history richly developed independently in an ancient and insular culture. Special doctors, who closely aligned cooking and medicine, herbalist pharmacists, and chefs combined the best of nutrition for the preventative care that still brings millions of people from both east and west to seek them out. Many philosophers, scholar gourmets, poets, and painters often treat food and drink as both the source and the subject of their work.

Food—its selection, preparation, and consumption—is a cause of harmony for the mind as well as for the senses. Decisions about a dish's ingredients depend on taste and texture, size and shape, and color and aroma, usually with an idea of balance or harmony, but sometimes honoring a single aspect of the palette.

Food is meant to be humanizing rather than brutish; that is one of the reasons chopsticks and porcelain spoons are used for eating while knives, cleavers, and forks are left in the kitchen.

Even the cuisine's famous five-spice blend serves a many-layered function. Five is a significantly potent number in China; the heavens are divided into five, and the five sacred mountains, Shantung, Hunan, Shensi, Ho-pei, and Honan are the pillars of China. The five virtues, the five tones, the five colors, and the five flavors are all benign and bring good fortune when used properly.

The wise and witty philosopher Chuang Tzu is most popularly known in the West for posing the question of whether he was a man dreaming he was a butterfly or having a butterfly's dream of being a man. In a poem he suggested that the emperor learn to be centered in his actions by watching his cook: "A good cook needs a new chopper once a year—he cuts. A bad cook needs a new one every month—he hacks."

All major traditions in China address the preparing and eating of food. In *The Confucian Analects* (Chapter VII), it was written about a virtuous person that:

1. He did not dislike to have his rice finely cleaned, nor to have his meat minced small.
2. He did not eat rice which had been injured by heat or damp and turned sour, nor fish nor flesh which was gone. He did not eat what was discolored, or of a bad flavor, nor anything which was ill cooked or not in season.
3. He did not eat meat which was not cut properly, nor that was served without its proper sauce.
4. Though there might be a large quantity of meat, he would not allow what he took to exceed the due proportion to the rice.
5. He was never without ginger when he ate.
6. Although his food might be coarse rice and vegetable soup, he would offer a little of it in sacrifice with a grave, respectful air.

Regional Cuisines of China

A variety of regional cuisines that were originally quite distinctive can be found in many large Chinese cities. In all regions soups with herbs, seeds, and roots are made, and sometimes several soups are served during a large meal. Appetizers or small dishes called *ping poon* start most formal meals. *Bat dai, bat siu* are meals of eight small cold dishes and eight large hot ones. *Congee*, a rice porridge (which I think will gain acceptance with increasing Western interest in healthy eating) is served like polenta with various savory or sometimes sweet accompaniments. *Fan*, virtually any carbohydrate, rice, grain, bread, or noodles, and *tsai*, fish, poultry, meat, or vegetables, are served in as many combinations as there are cooks, although certain dishes have been handed down in precise, unaltered, and ceremonial fashion for literally thousands of years.

In Guangzhou, the capital of Guangdong province (Canton) in the south, rice, vegetables, and fresh fish from its lengthy shoreline are steamed, blanched, or poached and frequently served with the simple addition of vinegar, ginger, scallions, and Chinese parsley. Soy, *hoisin*, and oyster sauces are among the traditional ones used. There are also many forms of barbecue or lacquer-roasted poultry and meat.

Steamed, baked, or fried dumplings, *dim sum* made of pork, beef, sausage, vegetables, sweet lotus, or bean paste, and spring rolls are sold everywhere, from street vendors to elegant tea houses. In large hotels and restaurants, elaborate food design results in sculpted presentations of a variety of foods to form a large butterfly or peacock, designed to elicit ooh's and ah's. By contrast, desserts are often simple sweet puddings, soups, or fruit.

Beijing in the north, once the seat of the imperial court and famous in the West for Peking duck, is not a rice region. Wheat prevails in noodles, dumplings, and bread. Duck and mutton or lamb are mainstays in the diet. Its hot pots, like fondue but using boiling water instead of oil, as well as casseroles and dramatic sizzling platters, are filling comfort foods for the cold winter months.

Shandong and Honan are included in what Westerners generally refer to as the "Mandarin" cuisine of the north. These regions were greatly influenced by Manchurian and Moslem cuisines and are famous for their aromatic lamb dishes. Some feast delicacies such as shark's fin soup and bird's nest soup originated elsewhere, but have long been elaborated on and served here.

Shanghai, the country's largest port, is in the northeast. In the fall the local crabs and their roe are so popular that visitors travel long distances to taste them. Currently Shanghai cooking is dominated by stir-frying with small quantities of meat or poultry and large amounts of fresh produce seasoned with sesame oil and soy sauce. The right *wok hay* (*wok* aroma) is the sign of a good cook. Often food is steamed and accompanied by preserved or pickled vegetables, depending on the season. Popular Shanghai cooking sometimes uses a lot of sugar and rice wine in sweet and sour dishes in which the meat or chicken is cooked for a long time.

Sichuan (Szechuan), modern China's largest province, is in the northwest and its eastern plains are among the most fertile in China. Barley, corn, fruit, potatoes, rice, sugar cane, vegetables, wheat, and tea are harvested here in abundance. Piquant and spicy dishes using onions, garlic, anise, ginger, chilies, and peppercorns are abundant. The chili peppers are an addition imported from the Mediterranean and are only a few hundred years old. Some local dishes are cooked with fresh flowers. Chicken and pork are used a great deal, as are sauteed vegetables. Sometimes the meat is smoked or barbecued. Wrapped dishes are popular as well; beanflour paste noodles, pancakes, and lotus leaves may all be used as wrappers. It is an overall complex flavor that Sichuan chefs strive for.

Adjacent Hunan province produces more fiery dishes than Sichuan and uses more game, such as venison and boar. This may explain why the people who live here use chopsticks half again as long as any found in Asia.

Sawaddi cuisine is vegetarian and designed for certain Buddhists and others who abstain from animal, fish, or egg protein. The Buddhist scripture *The Lotus Sutra* (250 B.C.E.) says:

> The rain, everywhere equal,
>   Descends equally on all four sides,
> Infusing without measure,
>   So that the whole earth is filled.
> The mountains', rivers', steep valleys',
>   And cavernous recesses' products of
> Grass, trees and medicinal herbs,
>   Of trees great and small,
> Of a hundred grains, of shoots and plants,
>   Of sweet potatoes and grapes,
> Infused by the rain,
>   Do not fail to prosper.

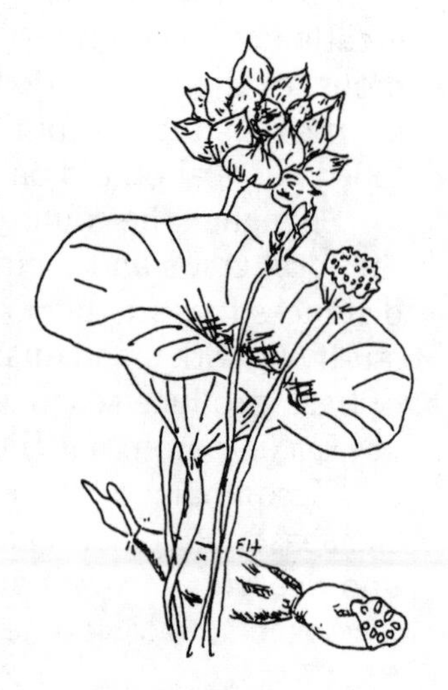

Lotus, Lotus Seeds, Lotus Root

1

CHINESE HISTORY

In China, people were cooking food when a good deal of the human race was still eating it raw. In 1000 B.C.E. a dietitian was appointed to the royal court, and recipes, with niceties like ginger and star anise, were drawn like poetry on silk scrolls. The scarcity of fuel led to elaborate preparation and efficient cooking time. Draft animals were used for work, not eating. Grain, rice, seeds, buds, and petals, as well as stems and leaves, were eaten for both philosophical and practical reasons.

China's varied geography—torrid rainforests, glacier caps, high peaks and valleys, wetlands, deserts, and lengthy coastline—is contained on a land mass only slightly larger than the United States and provides food for its citizens, who now number one-quarter of the world's people. China is bordered by mountains to the south and west, by the ocean to the east, and to the north, by the Great Wall, completed in the third century B.C.E. to hold the desert and invaders at bay.

For thousands of years, finely honed agricultural skills have sustained an ever-growing population with systems and principles that other countries are even now beginning to emulate, especially in the face of the failure of rampant technology to solve world hunger. With the development of irrigation systems, hill terracing, double cropping, the subordination of animals to crops, and methods of aquaculture or fish farming, food development has been an integral part of all activity in China for thousands of years. With primitive tools, agriculture was developed in the rich loess soil. Unsurprisingly, the major provinces of China are arable. Its most populous areas have always been labor-intensive agricultural domains.

Food culture is the basis of Chinese civilization. The early rulers of China assembled a workforce to cultivate, irrigate, harvest, and defend food supplies. Between 6000 and 5000 B.C.E., the beginnings of the farming that fed early civilization are visible in archeological artifacts, such as large storage pits for food, millet seeds, storage jars, choppers and hoes, sickles and shovels, millstones, chopping blocks, and mortars and pestles. In addition to agricultural tools, archeologists have also found bows and arrows for hunting; hooks, harpoons, and stone net-sinkers for fishing; and, of course, amphora. The early pottery, built from coils and smoothed, is said to have been fired at 900° to 1,000° C. Some of their neolithic linear designs and fish motifs have a surprisingly modern look. Between 4000 and 3000 B.C.E., farming communities proliferated. Archives from this period show bamboo shoots, grasses, chestnuts, pine nuts, and walnuts.

By 6000 B.C.E. there was millet, by 5000 B.C.E. there was rice, by 3000 B.C.E. there were vegetable gardens, and by 1000 B.C.E. soybeans were cultivated. By 1500 B.C.E. the Shang Dynasty (1766–1050 B.C.E.) had large cities and the first recorded cuisine. They dined on fish and poultry, as well as fruit and vegetables in and out of season, storing and preserving food by drying, pickling, and salting. The Yellow River valley was ruled by the Shang emperors who established water works and encouraged, supported, and rewarded agrarian prosperity.

Need drove both invention and an inventive art of cuisine that gave as much honor to the food of the common people as to the food on the emperor's table. Though the latter has always been more elaborate and extravagant than the former, the principles are the same. Every food and flavoring that came to China was given a chance to become part of its cuisine. If a plant could be cultivated, it was. Natural resources were quickly enhanced by imagination and not an edible morsel was left unused.

Historically there has always been an integration of nutrition, ritual, and medicine in China. When food is prepared, the cycle of the seasons is still given consideration as is the weather and the physical condition of family members. An internal or external change initiates a change in diet for a general or specific beneficial effect. Some combinations of ingredients are made into tonics that nourish and strengthen, prevent debilitation, or cure illness. Though most of these ingredients are plants, some are animal derivatives. Since China has strong personal and political disparities in its economy, traditional medical beliefs that encourage the use of natural resources give people a sense of dependability. Though some cures are fabulously expensive, most are quite modestly priced. Most are also high in nutrition and act as preventatives in many cases and as cures in others. In the West, *Rx* is Latin for "recipe" and "pharmaceutical prescription;" in Chinese the one word *fang* means formula for food or medicine.

Chinese street vendors have plied their skill and trade for a thousand years. In many areas one gets better food from food stalls and peddlers than from restaurants. In the second century B.C.E. a famous statesman and poet proposed "take-out" restaurants near the border of Mongolia to tame the "barbarians" who used their shields as grill plates and their sabers to cut and sometimes skewer meat over the fire. By the Tang Dynasty one could buy food, tea, wine, and snacks, until the small hours of the morning.

Today China still reaps the legacy of thousands of cooks and purveyors of food to both royalty and mendicants. Clearly the Silk Route was not only lined with bazaar items and religious shrines, but also with food stalls from every region. In all trading cities there is an ancient tradition of eating food from far-off places. Those who resettled brought culinary styles as well as spices and seeds from home. At Silk Route termini there was a need for food sources to be dependable, so that these places would be stable destinations for traders and benefit from regular business. This motivated communities to develop agriculture and cuisine that were available from year to year.

In the Han Dynasty (206 B.C.E.–220 C.E. (the Chinese people, unified, are known as "The People of the Han") capital of Ch'ang-an, now called Xi'an, texts and records show government interest in agriculture and public works, fertilizers, rice irrigation, storage pits, and crops and soil paired for quality. Iron tools were developed and ginger, litchis, lotus, melons, scallions, sesame, sugar cane, and honey flavored the ducks, geese, pheasants, and pigeons used in cooking. Pond carp as well as fish from native waters were cooked with herbs and other food-medicine. Using cormorants to fish was another early practice that continues today. Small ecosystems were created by leading ducks through rice fields to fatten themselves on insects, snails, and weeds. The ducks in turn fertilized the fields which were used to grow crops.

Major Chinese Provinces

Hunan Province

This province is now famous for being the birthplace of Mao Zedong, who was born in Shaoshan, a village about 60 miles southwest of Changsa, the capital. Mao was not adverse to gourmanderie and it is said that he so favored the hot taste of home that he had the bakers put chili peppers in his bread for the Long March.

Excavations of tombs at Mawangdui, just outside Changsa, show that among the beliefs of the early Han was the idea that humans are two souls joined in one body; *po* is the soul of the earth and will return to it after death, and *hun* is from the heavens and will ascend there at death. In the search for longevity, one elixir was taken to prevent the loss of the *po*, another to restrain the flight of the *hun*.

Found buried with the deceased, were not only texts such as the *Yiching* and Taoist breathing exercises but nourishment for the earthly soul: baskets of dried, salted, smoked, and pickled meat and fruit; pots of cereals, grains, vegetables, and cakes; jars of sauces, vinegar, and oil; and the favorite recipes of the departed. Traditionally, drawings of food were burned at interments and for several years after their demise the deceased were included in family feasts of the living.

Shandong Province

Shandong province, located on the eastern coast of China just north of Jiangsu, is famous for its seafood, braised meat, and poultry cooked in the subtle brown sauces that are the bases for most northern cuisine. Confucius (Kong Fuzi), born in Shandong in the sixth century B.C.E., wrote at length about food in season, healthy eating, and hygiene in the Analects (*Lun Yu*), which contain hundreds of food references.

Beijing, which became the capital of China in 1000 C.E., is generally considered to be in the Shandong food tradition, along with many Sichuan and Mongolian influences. Many food historians believe that Peking Man discovered cooking when he thawed frozen meat as he warmed himself by the fire. Marco Polo, who arrived at the end of the Sung Dynasty (960–1279 C.E.), writes of cities with large markets attracting as many as 50,000 people. He mentions potatoes, maize, and other New World crops as well as game, fish, fowl, fruit, vegetables, rice, and tea. He also describes meals of cabbage and cornmeal cakes, soups, and dumplings seasoned with ginger, brown pepper, cassia, and nutmeg.

The Ming Dynasty was established in Beijing. The first emperor of the Ming Dynasty (1368–1644 C.E.) was the descendant of farmers and he honored his common background. In a kitchen that served both the living and the deceased (at an inner temple called *feng xian tian*—"offerings for imperial forebears") chefs prepared fried cake, steamed bread, twice-cooked fish, honey cakes, pork, game, and rice and noodle dishes. The Ming Dynasty was also a time of art and science and the national palace known for centuries as the Forbidden City (*Jin Cheng*) was built during this period.

Through the royal courts of the Yuan (1264–1368), the Ming (1368–1644), and the Qing (1644–1911) Dynasties, northern cuisine was developed and refined. It was here that shark's fin soup and swallow's nests in consomme were and are served with such delicate dishes as oysters, conch, and sea cucumber in sauce. On the northern plains local crops include, in addition to wheat and millet, apples, cabbage, maize, sesame, peaches, peanuts, pears, peas, persimmons, plums, sesame, and sweet potatoes.

Sichuan Province

For more than 1,000 years, Sichuan province in the southwest of China has been known all over the world for its cuisine. With a population of more than 100 million people, Sichuan's kitchens are busy. In addition to various hot peppers, Sichuan black pepper or *fagara* is used to spice food, along with fermented black beans, sesame and bean pastes, garlic, ginger, scallions, soy sauce, and wine. One of the local favorites is *dan dan* noodles, which are flavored with dried shrimp, shredded preserved vegetables, peanuts, sesame seeds, chili oil, vinegar, and garlic. The other equally famous dish is *ma-po dofu*, red-hot bean curd stew. Chicken with peanuts in hot sauce, twice-cooked pork (boiled then fried), *bang bang* chicken (shredded chicken with a spicy sesame sauce), and "lampshade" beef (cooked in cellophane noodle pouches) are other popular dishes from this region.

The extra piquancy of Sichuan's food is famous, but now Guilin is becoming one of the major growers and packagers of various hot peppers and hot pepper sauces that are used internationally.

The need for Chinese restaurants in the United States to identify themselves with regional Chinese cuisines has caused a lot of confusion. When we set out to prove the geographical boundaries of these menu designations, it is quite difficult. Because of China's highly planned food systems there is some overlapping from province to province, although famous regional dishes are unique and memorable, like a song one can hum. Interestingly enough, these dishes tend to be quite forgiving in their preparation and in this way assure their longevity and reproducibility. Cultures and individuals tend to be traditional about food, and though dishes may change, their roots are respected.

Jiangsu Province

This province is perhaps less recognized outside of China than its better-known cities of Hangzhou, Nanjing, and Shanghai. This wealthy area is not only the land of rice and fish but, because of its location on the Grand Canal, has been influenced by northern, southern, and off-shore cultures. Completed during the Sui Dynasty (581–618 C.E.), the Grand Canal is the oldest and longest of its kind. It originally covered more than 1,000 miles, from Beijing to Hangzhou. Here both snacks and main dishes are well known. Steamed Mandarin fish and crab-roe dumplings are but two examples.

A representative of the Sheraton Hotel in Shanghai was recently kind enough to arrange for me a lunch at the Sheraton Huating and an interview with the deputy director of the Shanghai Municipal Tourism Administration. At lunch we ordered (I have steamed fish with ginger and vinegar, served with soup and rice) and then the director very kindly decided to share some of his knowledge of Chinese culinary history with me. He says:

> Of course, food and beverage is as long as the history of China; some historians say there are four main types, others say eight. There is an old saying, 'Along the moving of a stream—prosperity.' Without the water of the stream there is no prosperity. First prosperity, then moving ahead, development.

Of the four cuisines the first is the Lu cuisine of Shandong in the northeast. It follows the Yellow River. The second is Sichuan, at the upper part of the Yangtze. The third is the Hu, which is located on the flat plain at the lower level of the Yangtze. The fourth is the Yu or Cantonese. They are all related to water, as in the saying when you meet a stream, prosperity, then development. The Lu is the original cuisine of China; the Yellow River is the mother river. In modern history, cuisine is traced back only to Confucian culture, but it is actually pre-Confucian and after Shen Nung.

It is questionable that Lu cuisine is not considered important and that gourmets do not acknowledge early roots. They think of Lu as provincial food, but in earlier times it represented the whole area of the river. For those who believe there are eight basic types, the other four are the Xiang or Hunan, the Hui or Enhui, the Fujien or Ming, and ZeJiang Province. So it comes to the original saying. When you meet a stream, prosperity. When the water moves, there is development of the cuisines.

In the past ten years in Shanghai, Cantonese food has become popular, followed by Chaochou, and then Sichuan. Now the specific Shanghai cuisine is re-establishing itself and as it develops, Shanghai also develops cuisines from all over the world to please visitors and residents. They appreciate the promotion of Chinese food and the thousands of restaurants especially approved for tourists have high standards of skills in terms of dishes and food preparation.

There is a rating system for chefs. First is the senior executive chef, then the senior technical chef who is also a professor and enjoys academic status, and then there are categories of super chefs, who specialize in areas like eastern *dim sum* or western *dim sum*. There are also chefs who prepare the food of other cuisines, and there is a famous Chinese chef in Shanghai who can do French food. Along with development, food culture may be exchanged in a rapid manner and relationships are improved.

Guangdong Province

Guangzhou, which used to be known in the west as Canton, was for many years the prevailing place of birth for most of the Chinese that later settled in the West. The Hakka (a group originally from Keijia in the north that migrated hundreds of years ago) are usually figured in this category. As a result, the first restaurants they set up served the homey foods that would economically feed their community. *Chow mein*, variously sauteed noodle dishes, was a standby, as were egg *foo yung* and eggrolls. *Chop suey* was concocted in North America to use small bits of miscellaneous foods in a one-dish meal that could be cooked over little fuel and extended with rice. Some of the condiments everyone recognizes, such as plum sauce, oyster sauce, shrimp paste, fish extracts, and *satay*, are popular. *Dim sum* is a Cantonese institution and tea houses serve as places not only for *yum cha* but as meeting places for friends and family. Here business is conducted and a lone visitor can read the paper or write letters and never be rushed.

Cantonese chefs at home and abroad are great improvisers. It is said they will cook anything with four legs but the table. When one considers the floods and famines, invasions and epidemics, and wars and deprivations that have plagued their province, this approach seems very sensible.

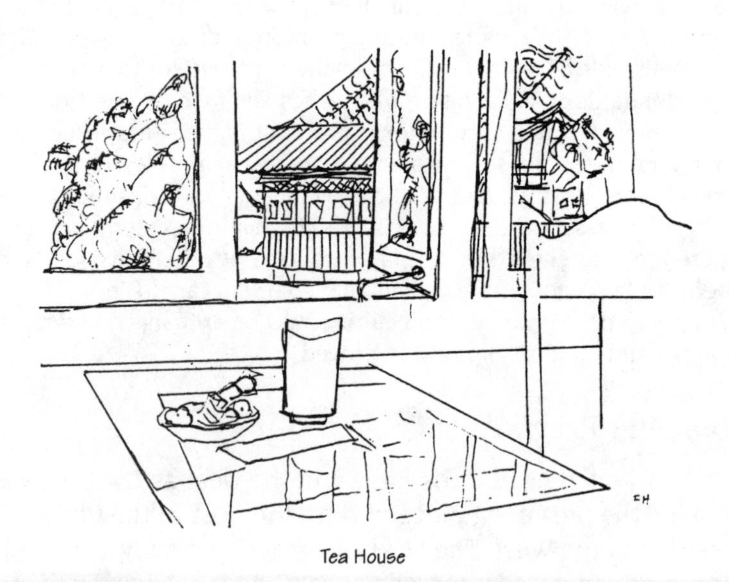

Tea House

2

FROM CHANG'AN INTO XI'AN

Sunday

In 194 B.C.E. Han Huidi built an imperial city called Chang'an, "Everlasting Peace." Now called Xi'an or "Western Peace," it is the largest city in northeast China, the capital of Shaanxi province, and has been populated for thousands of years. It is the eastern terminal of the Silk Road and was once the most important city in Asia. The Romans traded in its bazaars and Julius Caesar wore silk garments from China.

There are signs that since 6000 B.C.E. people in this area have irrigated the land, made dams, dug canals, cultivated millet and vegetables, and domesticated animals. Over time, projects have become larger in scale and now it is said that there is a "great wall" of greenness more than 200 miles long. Water conservation has allowed for terraced crop planting and now the Wei River valley produces a large amount of rice.

I arrive at the Sheraton Xi'an in a misty rain and, after settling in, call a taxi. It is after 7:00 P.M. on a rainy Sunday and I ask for Dong Dajie, a main avenue. We drive through the old city gate and to the Bell Tower after a night ride through streets still wet, but filled everywhere with street stalls and trestle tables set up for meals.

The driver parks near the Bell Tower Hotel to wait for me. I walk around in my relaxed dousing-method way and find a large dining hall with lots of long white tables spotted with hundreds of spilt soups and seating six to eight white slip-covered chairs. I walk in, starving, and the young women ask if I am alone, using one or two

English words, one or two Chinese words, and a lot of body language. I get a ticket for one order of dumplings and select my cold-plate assortment. The bill is 15 *yuan*, under two U.S. dollars.

I am seated casually at a table with one or two other singles. My cold plate has crisp sliced lotus and carrots, duck bits, bean curd slivers, and what appear to be long bean stems and yellow rice noodles. The dumplings are served in a great hot mound with a little bit of the broth they are boiled in. They are doughy and chewy like eastern European *pirogi* and are filled with vegetables, a small bit of meat and ginger, and a touch of coriander. The dipping sauce is vinegar, soy sauce, and chili flakes, which you compose from large serving containers on a tray in the middle of each table.

Later I find out that the place is well known and is the dumpling restaurant of the Defachang Hotel. It was awarded the Gold Tripod Prize by the Ministry of Commerce in 1989. I have eaten "1,000 year-old flavored boiled dumplings." It occurs to me that Xi'anese cooking is among the best of provincial cooking in China because a "people's" cuisine has been dominant for almost 1,000 years. The cuisine also benefits from the fact the flavors from along the trade route have mixed with those of neighboring regions and some, like curries, have become local dishes. The most ordinary food has a many-layered flavor structure: onions, garlics, leeks, shallots; fermented soybean sauces and pastes; vinegar and wine; and aromatic spices.

I walk around the Bell Tower a bit and people are out and about. There are always people out and about in China. Pedestrians, bicycles, cars, and buses move at a slower pace here than in Beijing. Dong Dajie is replete with hotels, shopping arcades, grocery stores, antique and dry goods shops, and department stores that carry everything from lingerie to electronic goods, household furnishings, solar panels, and satellite dishes. The restaurants vary from Mongolian Hotpot to Honey Hamburger.

Monday

Up early and eager to get out, I decide to eat breakfast in a lobby restaurant. I sit down in a comfortable armchair facing a wall of windows and order *congee*. It is delicious, a little soupier than I have had before, but hot and flavorful with good bits of pickle and smoked fish. Though there is a fine rain falling, people have stopped to do *tai ch'i* in the courtyard and along the street.

I meet with the hotel's executive chef, Raj Gupta, who has been around, from Delhi to Ayers Rock. He understands what it takes to get most Westerners to eat authentic Chinese food, and his breakfast buffets offer a large selection so that people can try new things with the security of knowing that they can have their familiar food as well. Tomorrow we will tour the Chinese kitchen and do a tasting. I ask about the stacks of corn on the cob layered straight up tall poles to dry that I have seen on the farms. This corn is used mainly for soup, not pastas or bread, he tells me. Cabbage, is dried in a similar way, with the leaves hung to dry in the sun for two or three months. Apples and other fruit are dried on rooftops.

I also explain that I hope that talking about Chinese food will make it more accessible to travelers and encourage joint ventures in China to help preserve it as well. There are already so many negative additions and substitutions to the local diet, such as white bread instead of whole wheat and even the disappearance of baked sweet potatoes as a street snack. All the good things in sweet potatoes—beta carotene, fiber, sugar, and of course their great taste on a cool afternoon—are being replaced by candy bars. I hate to think that in twenty years nutritionists will be advising people here against empty calories as they do in the States and will have to reteach diet and exercise as one of the main tools in avoiding preventable diseases.

I meet a translator and driver at noon and we proceed to the Tang Dynasty Training Institute and Restaurant.

During the rich cultural era of the Tang Dynasty, citizens were farmers, merchants, traders, scholars, and artisans. Works of gold, silver, and jade as well as silks and ceramics were exquisitely fashioned. Travelers from Byzantium, Arabia, Persia, Tibet, Burma, India, Korea, and Japan brought their culture and trade with them and took China's back. The Tang was a cosmopolitan golden age, and Chang'an was its capital. In Japan, Kyoto and Nara are modeled after it, as is Kyongju in Korea.

It was a very intellectual era and a time of prolific writing on all subjects, including food and cookery. Herbs and spices were enumerated and their aromatic and pharmaceutical properties described.

Cuisine and medicine were seen as working hand and hand. In the Tang, herbal pharmacologists codified the cool elements of Yin, the hot ones of Yang, and those that are neutral. It set standards for balance and harmony in food. Asparagus, cabbage, spinach, and turnips are cool, as is seafood. Chili, ginger, chicken, and lamb are among the hot foods. Rhubarb (*ta huang*) was highly regarded for digestion, though in modern times it is mainly an export and one of the few crops out of favor in China except in medicinal compounds.

In the Tang, tea became popular not only as a beverage but as an occasion for socializing. There were great varieties of dumplings, steamed bread, *wontons*, and sweet and savory buns and cakes to accompany it.

The Qu Jiang Chun restaurant is located on a busy street in a building it shares with a bank at 192 Jiefang Lu, which is also the proving ground for the institute.

On the building's third floor in the Concubine's Dining Chambers (*Yang Gui Fei*) are Lin Jianhua, an economist who is the restaurant's general manager as well as schoolmaster at the Institute, and Liu Jun Ling, the senior chef. We have tea from lacquered cups and begin to talk, starting with the concerns of research and preservation. Beginning with the names of dishes, ingredients, descriptions, and works of art, the Institute's chefs and researchers have tried to put together the court cuisine of the Tang Dynasty. In libraries they found some recipes and chef's notes as well as letters describing meals.

The school was opened in 1982 and trains 700–800 chefs every year. They are mainly men, though they say there is no prohibition against women. They explain that Western people are usually only interested in the exotica, like camel's foot soup. I tell them I understand; in Egypt I have seen camels marked for slaughter being led through the streets. In an arid region there are no fish or fowl or, for that matter, much of anything; within that context the camel is a logical food source.

They give me some photos and inscribe their book to me. Ready for a photo opportunity, we walk through the restaurant's three floors, including the Emperor's Dining Hall, with its dragon mural and the room for ordinary people, the name for which they give as *Zhui Xian*.

I have been promised "ordinary" *Xué mian* (yes, *chow mein*) so we go to Dao Xue' Mian on Tumen Dajie. In the street, over an open fire, the noodles are cooked in a great *wok* with some bean sprouts, ground pork, *ching cai*, ginger, coriander, and a brown gravy. On the table are mayonnaise jars filled with soy sauce or vinegar, an uncovered cup of ground red chilies, and a plastic tub of raw garlic cloves. It is hot and delicious. We are served the cooking broth as soup in a small bowl. I am warm and full. The bill for the two of us is four *yuan*, or about fifty cents.

I head for the Shaanxi History Museum, that was opened in 1991 and is wonderfully modern, though architecturally in the style of the Tang Dynasty. Using *feng shui*, it emphasizes harmony along an axle, yet its installation and preservation techniques are advanced, with temperature and humidity control run by computers. In the auditorium most functions and events are simultaneously translated into six languages. The collection of almost half a million objects is archived, preserved, and stored with the aid of twenty-first-century behind-the-scene operations. Though true to the new low-tech entrepreneurial spirit, the museum is filled with seemingly independent vendors selling competitively the items one finds in museum shops. They follow you into the galleries, hawking their wares *sotto voce*.

The collection includes gold, silver, and jade wares; porcelains; glass; and tableware of great variety. One can also see bronze pots and cooking vessels, kettles, and jars that are sculpted and incised with great skill and beauty.

The Shaanxi History Museum is built on the site of a fourteenth-century Confucian temple and in addition to the archival collection, there is the forest of stele. Inscribed on many stele are the stories of diverse religions, including Christianity, which was present during the Tang Dynasty for 200 years. Though Confucianism was the austere state doctrine, it existed without a hierarchical organization. A medley of beliefs co-existed quite harmoniously; there were times of great turbulence, it was rarely over doctrine. Confucian, Taoist, Lamaist, and Buddhist temples, as well as a still-active eighth-century mosque, reflect the many beliefs that have nourished the Chinese population.

Xi'an has a large Muslim population and there are many street markets that sell ethnic food and crafts. *Pao mo* is the dish I want, as I have never had it before. There is a tourist *pao mo* restaurant that is on everyone's itinerary, but I ask for the place where the locals eat. A secretary at the Sheraton writes the name of another restaurant that she likes in Chinese, so I can give it to the cab driver. I set out with a driver who has a buddy accompanying him, and the two are singing along to pop songs on the radio. It is great, except they cannot find the place and we have to ask several people before we get there. Finally we find it on the corner of a main street, around the corner from the Great Bell Hotel and down about ten or twelve blocks.

In the *Lao Sun Jia Pao Mo* Restaurant, I am on my own and no one speaks a word of English. There are only a handful of people eating in the restaurant. I go to the cashier and bread server and ask for an order of *pao mo*. She hands me the thick pita-like bread, a bowl, a pair of chopsticks, and two small dishes—one with cooked garlic cloves and the other with minced red pepper. I know I am supposed to tear the bread and put it into the bowl, but I am not making the pieces small enough to suit the cashier, so she starts to help me. Soon another server comes over and the three of us are making minced bread. They motion me to sit down. I take out the note that has brought me there and, with two or three Chinese words, tell them how I was told this was a very good place. We all smile. They take the bowl and ask me into the kitchen. The chefs are having a good time and one in a fez asks to take a picture with me. Of course I comply. For this old style Yangrou *pao mo*, bowls are filled with torn bits of spongy flat bread, then cooked with lamb soup, usually a mixture of tomatoes, bean threads, scallions, and minced or diced roast lamb seasoned with anise, cinnamon, ginger, soy sauce, and chili paste. It has the consistency of western chili and it tastes almost familiar.

As I eat, different people come around and use my dictionary. One person in particular tries to talk with me and we more or less communicate. She asks what I do and tells me she thought I was Canadian. She says she is surprised I am American because she never sees Americans alone. Another woman, a customer, comes over and practices her English. We are having fun and I am eating my *pao mo* all the while, as I am really hungry. They explain that they want me to send them a couple of pictures and write the address for me. Afterwards, I take a long walk, enjoying my night-time freedom, and finally taxi back.

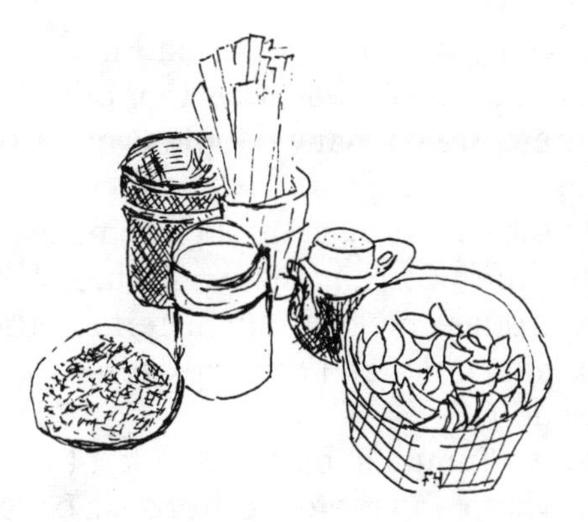

Condiments at Street Stall

Tuesday

I have a full Chinese breakfast downstairs and leave at 8:30 for the tombs. I know I have grown relaxed, since streets and streets of food stalls now seem ordinary neighborhood sights. As we drive through thriving farm country that looks a bit like eastern Long Island, the sun is quite spectacular as it emerges after three days of rain.

At the tombs there is a long avenue of vendors, as if for a festival. They are selling furs from the north, large baskets, bronzes, embroidered red cotton quilts, and clothing, both old and new, including children's vests and shoes decorated with animals and symbols to protect and keep them from harm. I buy more of them than I should. The food is abundant. The noodle makers are like a magic show. There are two principal ways noodles are made: one is pulled and stretched and twisted long, sort of like pulling taffy; the other is to take a great mass of dough and slice it as it is held high up in the air, straight into a pot of boiling water.

The Qin tombs are astonishing. As you approach one of three buildings that look like enormous airplane hangars, there is no clue of the sight to come. Called by some "the eighth wonder of the world," these are the tombs of soldiers of the Qin Dynasty. It is sobering—their faces are so touching, so beautiful, that I would love to be able to walk around them and to feel what they are feeling.

They radiate emotion and intelligence and not one face is like another. There are well designed walkways that bring you fairly close to the tombs, but there are so many people even at this hour that we must keep moving.

On the way to the car I browse through some of the stalls and buy some antique children's costume hats and three fake jade geese. At the gate someone offers me four small terra cotta warriors and a horse for one American dollar. I can't resist and will see if they get back intact. (They do.)

We drive then to Tumulus, burial mound of the Qin emperor. It has not been excavated and there are steps six or seven stories high straight up the face of it. I start first along the wall, where there are vendors of folk art, reproductions, handicrafts, and food. Every ten feet men and women of all ages are selling hot baked sweet potatoes, persimmons, apples, pomegranates, hot hard-boiled eggs, all the way up to the top where there is a small plateau, with people selling there as well. I buy a small brass *Kuan Yin*.

The young Emperor Qin Shi Huang Di, who reigned from the age of thirteen to twenty-five (221–209 B.C.), was the first emperor (*huang di* means emperor) of unified China in 221 B.C. He initiated the end of serfdom and brought fiefs directly under the law of the emperor. He standardized a system of money and weights and measures and, more importantly, unified the Chinese written language. He was cruel and despotic—not satisfied by burning books and inflicting cruel punishment, Qin Shi buried alive his intellectual enemies because he saw "dangerous thought" as the enemy of his dream. In his short reign, perhaps ten percent of the population was engaged in forced labor, the products of which were the Great Wall, the E'fang Palace, and the mausoleum and pits that contain the extraordinary subterranean army of 8,000 terra cotta soldiers, along with their horses and chariots.

As we leave, we pass the tourist restaurants, all with large buses parked outside them. This is Xi'an's major industry. I would like to stop and see what's going on, as they are enormous and quite elaborately decorated on the outside, but have other commitments.

My next stop is at the Banpo Museum, which is on the site of a neolithic village that was unearthed in 1953. Among the first discoveries were Stone Age millet and cabbage in storage jars from individual to community size, along with shovels, sickles, hoes, choppers, chopping blocks, and small and large millstones. There are also bows and arrows for hunting and hooks, harpoons, and stone net sinkers for fishing. Cookware included bowls, amphora, urns, jars, and pots, some with steamers made of clay. The Chinese had clay steamers at a time in history when some cultures did not even have clay pots! Most of the pottery is built up of coils, with the surface smoothed. The pottery is estimated to have been baked at 900° to 1,000° C. It was often decorated with stylized black fish over the reddish terra cotta, and some pieces are rough and decorated by fingernail incisions.

Next, off to a 3:00 tasting meeting with the general manager of the hotel, the executive chef, and the head Chinese chef. The cold plate is composed of thinly sliced five-flavor beef, barbecued pork (made in the traditional way: marinated, then roasted hung in a Chinese oven), and pork knuckle boiled in marinade, refrigerated three days, then thinly sliced. This is served with a honey, Sichuan pepper, and flaked red pepper dip on a plate with a white radish flower that has been done in silhouette. Next comes Xingin beef in an egg-noodle basket. A ring of rice is set on the plate and a fried noodle basket is set on the ring and filled. The filling is a layer of sauteed red onions cut in crescents, carrots cut into stars, and sweet peppers topped with tender slices of beef seasoned with cumin and chili peppers, in the local style. It is garnished with sprigs of coriander.

The next dish, Xianese sweet-and-sour carp, is made from fillets cut in slices to the skin in one diagonal, then in the other. The fillets are dipped in a batter of cornflour and egg, then deep fried. The sweet-and-sour sauce is flavored locally with the addition of chilies and pineapple. In most of China, sweet-and-sour sauces are for fish; meat and poultry are almost never served with it.

Our pork dumpling soup has a base of pork stock seasoned with chili, cumin, and oyster and soy sauces. Carrot, cabbage, celery, capsicums, and whatever vegetables are available are sliced thinly into the broth, which is then thickened with cornstarch in cold water. The small pork dumplings are made from lean pork finely ground with ginger, onion, chili powder, and cumin and rolled in cornstarch. They are first fried then simmered in the soup so they do not taste fried.

The dessert is a version of eight-flavor rice. Local short-grained rice is cooked with dates, raisins, cherries, almonds, pine nuts, and orange and tangerine peels. It is served unconventionally in a strawberry coulis.

The Empress Court Restaurant at the Sheraton Xian is wonderful. Dinner at the restaurant includes green tea shrimp, broccoli, and a grape wine tasting. The Dynasty Red is quite good.

Wednesday

After breakfast in my room, I go to the Big Wild Goose Pagoda (Temple of Great Goodwill) and then the Little Goose Pagoda. Legend has it that as a large wild goose flew over the site of the big pagoda it fell down dead. It was seen to be so beautiful and startling an event that the citizens thought a saint had come to earth. They built a temple on the spot to honor him. As people have done for 1,300 years, I climb to the top, up a steep angled spiral stair. It feels somehow like a pilgrimage, so I light candles and incense because it would feel strange not to. This brick and wood seven-story tower was originally built in 652 C.E., but was rebuilt between 701 and 704 C.E. It is this structure that still houses Buddhist transcripts and art. Not only is it structurally sound, but it looks precisely like the pagodas of our story books: seven stories, each stepped back, with details appearing as an imitation of wooden construction. The grounds have been recently refurbished and they are very pleasant to walk around. There are Tang Dynasty tablets describing Xuan Zang's journey to bring Buddhism to China, famously fictionalized in "Monkey," and ancient calligraphic graffiti. He returned with almost 1,000 Buddhist *sutras*, statues of wood, gold, and silver, as well as pieces of the Buddha's chair. There are also funeral *stupas* of sober beauty. Outside the walls there are food and art vendors, the latter selling everything from folk art to rubbings. I quickly realize that most of the pieces are skillful reproductions.

The vendors are selling eighteen-inch-long twisted noodles that are fried and left to harden. They are cold, a bit greasy and chewy, but very entertaining. I know I am being overcharged at one *yuan*.

Originally built as a fireproof storehouse for Buddhist *sutras*, the Little Goose Pagoda in the Temple of Commending Happiness is a stepped-brick pagoda. It is fine from the outside, but the greatest architectural interest is the inside, where the brickwork forms wonderful structural designs.

On its grounds are fruit sellers, a tea shop, and an art studio. I go inside the studio and wander to the back where a painter is mixing powdered pigment with glue (mucilage) and water. With a very fine brush he applies color to preprinted outlines. It looks like fun. As soon as I show interest, the big dictionary comes out and we try to talk. I am led further back into the studio, which contains rougher freehand work and heaps of discarded paint tubes for recycling. I leave and two young women stop and invite me to bang a large temple drum. They encourage me to get louder and louder and take my camera to snap me doing it. The loud clear tones they tell me are for a safe journey, a safe return. They say the word "safe" as though it were the word for "happy."

I take a cab to the airport by myself. The airport is very user-friendly—I am able to get an earlier flight than the one I booked and wander around while I wait. There are several restaurants and food vendors. Carts serve packaged "noodles in a cup." When purchased, the vendor fills the cup with hot water and offers a great wedge of sponge cake as well. There are also stands of free hot and cold water. A lot of people carry covered mayonnaise jars of tea from which they drink from time to time. Many are carrying baskets of persimmons as gifts to their destination. Everyone is talking but not frenetically. There is (surprisingly) no smoking permitted.

This is the first flight on which I may be the only one to speak English as a first language, but I am always amazed at how well one can manage if there is accord.

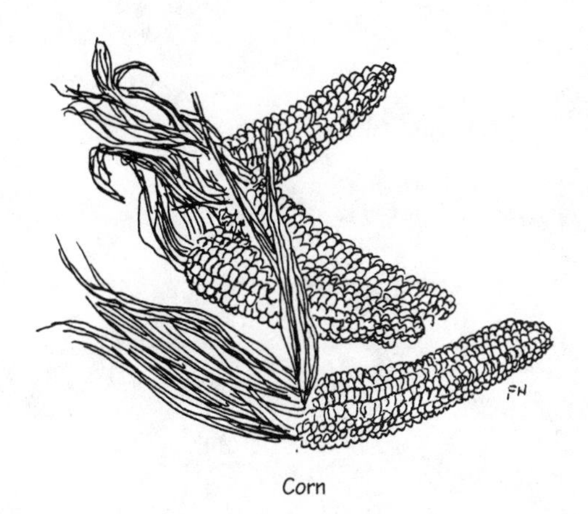

Corn

3

BEIJING AND THE NORTH

Monday

Getting from the plane and going through the airport is easy and casual, even though there are no signs in English about passport control, changing money, etc. The great bustle at the airport has a surprisingly familiar feeling. As I am about to get out my phrase book, I spot a representative from the Sheraton Great Wall Hotel who accompanies me to a cab, tells me what it should cost, and tells the driver to wait for me while I change money in the hotel. What a smooth transition for someone traveling alone!

The hotel is made of dazzling glass and steel. Its atriums, elevators, restaurants, shops, and business centers buzz. There is a large garden in the traditional Chinese manner with bamboo and regional plants, stone sculpture, footpaths with changing views, stepping stones over brooks, and a pavilion. Best of all, my room has every amenity.

Here I am in Beijing, or Peking, the ancient capital of Cathay, and I have a rush of feeling for the stuff of children's books. In the Qin Dynasty (221–206 B.C.E.) a city existed more or less where modern Beijing is. It was called Yanjing or the "Swallow Capital" because of all the swallows that to this day nest in the eaves of its buildings, old and new. Even at that time it was a large market and traded with places as far away as Korea.

When the troops led by Ghengis Khan overwhelmed China, Ghengis Khan moved the capital to this site and established the Yuan Dynasty (1264–1368 A.D.). In 1215 the city was named Khanbalik, or

"City of the Khan." During this era, Khan rulers dominated from the Pacific to the Danube.

Even before Marco Polo arrived in 1271, medieval travelers reported that the city's streets were laid out at right angles to each other and filled with stalls and shops, much like modern cities. Marco Polo wrote not only of the court of Kublai Khan, but of the merits of its cuisine and wine and of its doctors' knowledge of the effects of herbs and their ability to diagnose ailments by one's pulse. He describes how bamboo shoots were eaten like asparagus, and, in addition to other fruits and vegetables, remarks on barley, beans, chestnuts, ginger, ginseng, lentils, millet, oats, sorghum, walnuts, and wheat. He traveled widely and though some of his charts were wrong, he placed "Cathay" on the map of the known world. China was known to the West as Cathay for about 200 years. This error occurred because of an alternate pronunciation during the Mongol court. In 1607, Matteo Ricci, a Jesuit missionary, reported that Cathay and China were one and the same, and the name Cathay fell into disuse.

I am somehow compelled to go first to Tianamen Square where the Gate of Heavenly Peace was built in 1651, and since that time pronouncements of importance to the nation have been read from its balustrade. On October 1, 1949 Chairman Mao Zedong announced the establishment of the People's Republic of China. As a result, it is the only place there is a public portrait of the Chairman. The square is perhaps the most photographed place in modern China, since it has been the viewing area for all major public political displays. On June 4, 1989 the world watched as students and citizens peacefully demonstrating in support of greater freedom were dispersed by armed militia. Now, five years later, one senses some progress and a level of individual optimism that is very touching.

I am embarrassed that I find Tianamen Square exhilarating; it is filled with people walking, talking, and posing for pictures. They exchange cameras, even with me, and some want to be in the pictures with me. There are flower sculptures and playful fountains from the recent October 1 celebration. The level of energy is contagious. I walk around until almost dark. Only when I get back to the hotel do I realize how unusual it is to see someone alone here, especially a Western woman.

The Yuen Tai is a pretty restaurant with windows on all sides. I get some Shaoxing wine and am served delicious assorted pickles with it. For dinner I order eel and garlic, stir-fried vegetables, which are served with three kinds of peppers, a small hot and sour soup, and for dessert sweet *lai* dumplings, small sugar-filled dumplings in plain broth. The tea master is excellent. The cart has ceramic caddies (from the Chinese word *Catty*, which is the weight measure equivalent of 1.33 pounds) from which the tea is spooned into traditional covered cups; water is then added from a copper kettle held a few feet above the cup.

After dinner I go for a walk, first in the hotel, browsing through the "Silk Road" shops and bookstore. Then I go out. The only place to walk (except the highway) is past the New Park Towers and The Hard Rock Cafe, which has crowds of well-dressed young Beijingers waiting to get in. As in Western cities, there are aggressive beggars, some with children. The Lufthansa Center is a modern mall with expensive international merchandise such as jewelry, electronics, fashion clothing, and children's toys. Bottled water, packaged conveniences, sweets, and fresh cooked food are available. Outside there are foodstalls selling noodles and dumplings.

Finally, ready to call it a night, I go to my room. I shower and, in my robe, I channel surf. Marlon Brando is on "Larry King Live." I am having a complementary Martell VS cognac and a dark chocolate Dove Bar made in China. Nothing has prepared me for Beijing 1994. It is hurtling into the twenty-first century, but my education and aesthetics are more familiar with Buddhist temples and the starry sky.

Tuesday

I buy a flimsy green silk scarf with line-drawn trees. Now when I arrange to meet strangers, I can say I will be wearing a green scarf.

I spend the morning working and have a light lunch. Then, as arranged, I meet a friend, a Beijinger, and we go to the National Palace Museum, walking around and talking about how rapidly things are changing. We take a cab to the Palace Museum and the traffic and sights en route hold our attention and conversation. Actually seeing McDonald's, Kentucky Fried Chicken, and Baskin Robbins franchises takes a while to absorb. The numbers of people everywhere make me think that those scenes in movies that look like great exoduses scenes are merely depictions of rush hours. Vehicles of every description fill the streets. Women pedal bikes while wearing pumps. Everyone I see is well dressed. There are gates along the sidewalks, and you may have to walk blocks to get to where you can even cross the street or drive half a mile to make a U turn. There is construction everywhere. Old and new buildings stand side by side, and except for valued sites, no edifice seems to get repaired. Anything that is broken is not fixed but knocked down, and something very new takes its place.

The Ming Dynasty (1368–1644) began with its capital in Nanjing, but scholars and geomancers advised that the *feng shui* was better in Beijing and the capital was returned there in 1402. The 9,000-room Palace Museum covers 178 acres and was built from 1406–1420 to be the Imperial Palace of the Ming emperors.

Its walls are red, and the yellow color of the roof tiles that cover all the structures was permitted only to royalty. It is no longer considered correct to call the palace the "Forbidden City" (Jin Cheng). The "Last Emperor," Henry Aisin-Gioro Pu Yi (1906–1967), lived here as emperor from the age of two, but the last despot to reign was the Dowager Empress Cixi, whose power was of mythic proportion.

My friend buys two tickets, then we are told at the museum's gate that one ticket must be returned and another bought for me (at a higher rate) from a different window for tourists. My friend is surprised and comments upon how many things have changed.

We walk around the museum which, though it is filled with tourists from everywhere, is surprisingly quiet. Everyone stops and stares during walks across courtyard after courtyard, down walled alleys, and through small and large chambers, court rooms, seal rooms, and banquet halls; there are wonderful details everywhere. One can read many accounts of the history, art, and architecture of this complex, but actually to be here changes one's sense of the physical world.

There were complex food rituals in the court. The emperor did not decide the menu, so no one knew beforehand what was to be eaten. Decisions were made in the kitchen where there were one hundred stoves, each numbered. Written records were kept detailing which person was at each kitchen station and precisely what passed through their hands. At table the emperor never ate more than two portions of any dish, lest it be construed as a favorite and a potential one for enemies to poison.

We cannot enter any of the rooms because after Bertolucci's "The Last Emperor" was filmed the curators wanted to stem the damage caused by the crew and its equipment. The flower gardens, trees, stone mosaic pathways, rock gardens, and small pavillions invite strolling. Beijing is so rich in both historic and modern places of interest—landmarks, museums, temples, libraries, universities, individual houses, and mansions, as well as the restored observatory of Kublai Khan—that it would take ages to explore and enjoy.

For dinner my friend suggests that we go to a very famous Peking roast duck restaurant (Quanjude on Hepingmen), the original of which was established in 1864. This restaurant, now one of three in Beijing, has fifty satellite restaurants throughout China. Their repertoire includes 400 duck recipes, one hundred of which are used regularly. The most popular recipe is still the one in which the duck is eaten with flat pancakes, scallions, and sweetened bean sauce. The restaurant's "All Duck Banquet" may have as many as thirty duck courses, including crystal duck tongues, fried liver and gizzard, stew, and soups. It is as popular among Beijingers as it is with tourists. The restaurant was opened in 1864 by a duck farmer from Hebei Province named Quanren Yung. *Quanjude* is an anagram of *Dejuquan*, which was the name of the shop he took over for his restaurant. He served only duck dishes, and the style he developed has become a world-class treat. Shoubein Chen is now the restaurant's chief chef; he has been with them for forty years and says he knows 500 recipes by heart.

It is 6:00 and already the first three floors of public space and private dining rooms are full. We are the first, and for about ten minutes, the only ones in the fourth-floor ballroom of a dining hall with about fifty tables. My host suggests half a duck and two additional dishes and will not consider less. Sadly, we are both disappointed; the food is tepid, the duck's skin is greasy and not crisp, the pancakes are drying at the edges, and the scallions limp. Surprisingly, the soup is creamy and delicious. However, we are enjoying ourselves. In minutes the room fills to capacity. Everyone orders duck, and almost everyone photographs each other eating it amidst the large murals and painted masks from traditional characters in Chinese opera. The restaurant seats 2,500 people. It seems that everyone is eating and taking pictures of each other. I have long stopped being shy with my camera since everyone else seems so unembarrassed to be on either side of a lens. They make it very comfortable.

We walk after dinner and I comment on the crowds. My friend smilingly reminds me that there are even larger crowds indoors. Food stalls and markets are active and the streets are very lively. One neighborhood group is having a dance.

Back at the Sheraton, I sort the inks, brushes, ink stones, pigment, and paper I bought at Rong Bao Zhai on Liulichang. Since the early Qing Dynasty (1644–1911), this market street has been selling art supplies, as well as books, scrolls, fans, lanterns, tiles, and reproductions. Liulichang's historic appearance has remained intact thanks to preservation and restoration.

Wednesday

I am having lunch at the Yuen Tai restaurant on the twenty-first floor of the Sheraton. Everywhere on the horizon large mechanical cranes attest to the amount of building going on.

We go to the kitchen, which is modern and well designed. The chef is from Sichuan and uses something like a *tandoori* oven over which he handles the *wok*. He pours in the oil, swirls it to coat the *wok*,

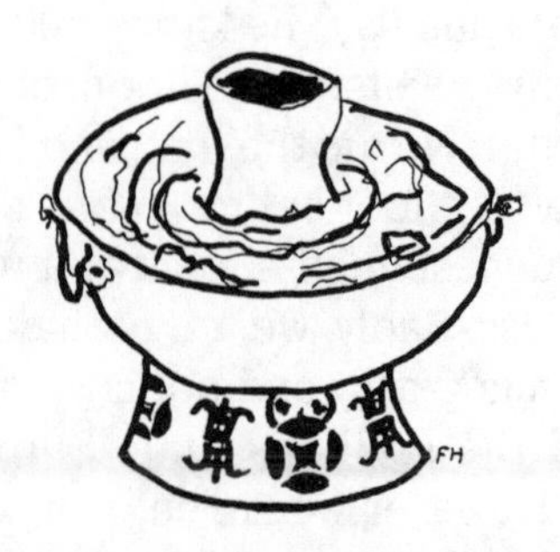

Mongolian Hot Pot

pours it out, and returns a small amount to coat the bottom of the *wok*. The chef then takes shoestring slices of pork and dusts them with cornstarch. He then stirs them into the *wok* with soy sauce, sugar, vinegar, sesame oil, and crushed Sichuan and chili peppers; he then adds slivers of ginger, onion, mushrooms, and bamboo shoots. The dish is quickly plated with a large radish flower and placed on a decorative metal collar so that the plate does not touch the cold table top.

We return to our table and are also served soup, a vegetable dish, and *dan dan* noodles. I have been drinking green tea, which the tea master makes from his wheeled cart. With our dessert of a cereal-textured custard with crumbled walnuts we have eight treasure tea. Added to the tea's mix of walnuts, raisins, dates, tiny plums, and cassia are tiny bright red wolfberries (*gouqizi.*) They are a little larger than holly berries, oval and wrinkled, soft and very tasty, somewhat similar to dried cranberries, but not as sweet as dried cherries. At first the tea does not taste sweet, but as second and third refills of hot water are poured over it, the sweetness emerges.

I spend the rest of the afternoon arranging travel plans, making phone calls, and taking care of other business. As a treat, I leave the hotel in the evening with a map and a dictionary and take a taxi to areas I have heard about. The driver is up for it and we take the scenic route along Embassy Row and some Chinese residences. We then visit a small local night market, badly lit. I get out and walk a block on each side, stopping to go into a crowded dry goods store, much like an old-fashioned "five and ten." I buy some whole wheat buns with sesame seeds from a woman baking them on a metal drum. I know that these will disappear and next year they will be made of white flour, though this is a wheat area, just as it was millet earlier. Progress changes cuisine, and some would say cuisine changes progress. I offer some to the driver, who says he doesn't like them.

We drive further and I stop at a bakery and an herbal medicine store standing side by side. At the bakery I buy a starfish-shaped sponge cake the size of a small hand that is decorated with a red seal, two walnut moon cakes, a fig cake, a chestnut bun, and a pretty round cake that tastes like fig. The driver likes these.

We drive along to the Dongdan Market and stop at a small department store that has no name in English. I get out and since the driver cannot park, he leaves me on my own. The store is crowded, as

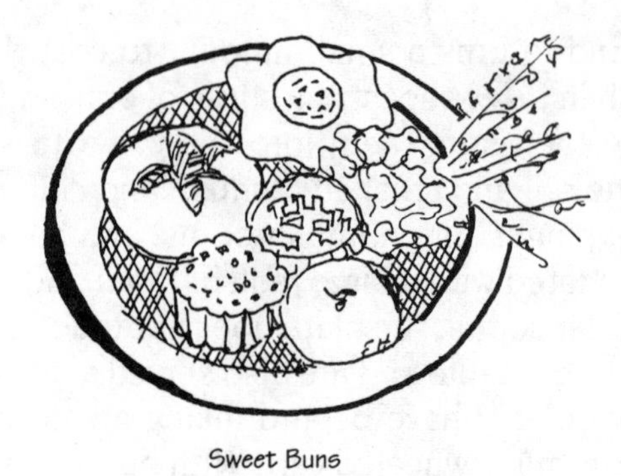

Sweet Buns

are the streets. Most public places and tourist attractions cannot be entered after 4:00, but here there is activity until well into the night .

Thursday

In the morning I make some calls and go to the China Art Gallery. The exhibit there is mainly a folk art show, very lively and quite interesting. As with some processes, watching people at work can be far more fascinating than the work itself. Artists are often great communicators (even when negative) because they frequently feel marginalized. I watch as woodblocks are cut and carvings, quilts, and models are made. I exchange hellos with some of the artists. One introduces me to someone from the Ministry of Culture who speaks English and we have a good talk. In the well-stocked book and supply store that seems run by and for students, I buy some how-to-paint-Chinese-fruits-and-vegetables books, as well as a sketchbook so fancy I will never use it.

I walk south towards the Beijing Hotel for lunch with someone from Boeing to whom I have an introduction. Her office is on the fifteenth floor and out the balcony window is the view we always see when we see news from China—all of Tiananmen Square and part of the Palace Museum. She sees the look in my eye and has seen it before, saying she will take my picture on the balcony. I say, "Of course."

Then, on the way to the Sichuan Restaurant in the hotel, I look around. The center of the building was built in 1917, one wing in 1954, then more wings in 1974. Its location has made it the place from which journalists have reported for almost eighty years.

We order vegetable dumplings served with a great vinegar sauce, fried prawns in spicy fruit sauce, and a seafood soup. Dessert is fried sweet dumplings and an undistinguished tea. We talk about life as single parents in Beijing, New York, and Seattle.

After lunch I walk along Jianguomen Dajie to meet with a journalist from Baltimore. We meet in front of the Friendship Store at the lion statue nearest Baskin Robbins. He arrives by bike and we walk back to his office a block or so away. He has been in Beijing a while and speaks Chinese fluently. He helps me understand that the experience I sometimes have in this city—of hearing a "yes" and then having nothing happen—is quite usual. I am, in fact, happy to hear that he thinks I am doing well to be getting accomplished even eighty percent of what I arrange. All professionals learn to negotiate "no" and its varying degrees, but this is the first city in my experience where "yes" has so many meanings. We have tea and a good talk about food and the importance it continues to play in all social encounters.

Back at the Sheraton, I pick up my new business cards that have my name rendered somehow also in Chinese. Everyone exchanges cards here. Then I meet Yan Zhen Cui, the deputy public relations manager at the Fortune Restaurant. She introduces me to Liang Xiao Qing, the Chinese kitchen executive chef from Beijing. He first started cooking Sichuan food, but is now in charge of the Yuan Tai Restaurant also. Dinner is *Chiu Chow* style. I have some warm Shaoxing wine followed by slices of goose and *dofu* served with a side sauce of white vinegar with bits of pepper and ginger I know the shark's fin soup is going to be good. It is served in tubs with lids to keep it hot and tasty and accompanied by dark vinegar. Next we have variously shaped fried shrimp balls with a sweet sauce, giant whole prawns with a bean sauce, chicken tidbits in fried potato baskets, and kale (spoon vegetable) braised with mushrooms. Dessert is assorted small sweet dumplings, two kinds of beans (a red and a brown) in transparent rice flour dough skins, and fried sesame balls. I enjoy both the dinner and the conversation very much.

Friday

After a very early breakfast of *congee*, fruit, and tea, I look through papers and notes and then have a swim and a sauna until it is time to meet a journalist from New York, who has been kind enough to come to my rescue when I say I haven't found a wonderful, ordinary restaurant.

We meet at the lion statue in front of the Friendship Store, *the* place for foreigners to meet. He brings a friend who is also a journalist. I am so pleased they have made the time for this. We take a cab to the front of the China Art Gallery on Jingshan Qianjie; the driver asks where we are going and, when told, says we have chosen the best restaurant in the neighborhood. We cross the street, make a right, walk past the public toilets, and then turn left at the first alley. In the middle of the block on the right-hand side is a sign with a multi-colored plastic strip curtain to guard against the flies. We enter a dark green room with about ten tables, quite crowded, the tables heaped high with dishes. We are lucky and instantly a table opens up. The menu is in Chinese characters only, which my companions read fluently. The name of the place is Joy Guest Restaurant, it is more or less Fanguanese, and it has been there quite a while. The chef's father cooked for Mao.

My host mentions a dish he likes called *yu xi'ang qie zi* (smells-like-fish-eggplant), which is sliced Chinese eggplant cooked with pork and chili peppers. Our orders start arriving: first, *wu tou*, an egg pancake rolled around five (*wu*) ingredients—duck, mushrooms, bamboo shoots, scallions, and something crisp. The rolls are served sliced with small hot pancakes, a thin spicy bean sauce, and scallion strips. It's delicious. We then get *xi'ang su yu qui*, Changsu fish chunks with a vinegar taste. Small pieces of freshwater fish are dipped in a vinegar and taro batter, lightly fried, and served so hot there is no oil at all. Just flavor. Then comes *ba bai ci*, cabbage leaves stewed with *dofu* skins that have been rolled a bit, like a scrambled egg. D*ofu he—dofu* with something involved—turns out to be a favorite—minced meat stuffed into flat squares of *dofu*, fried and sauced Sichuan style with bits of red pepper. Hot and aromatic, the texture is perfect. H*e lan dou*, or Holland peas look like pea pods to me and are fresh, crisp, and plentiful. *Jin qian rou* means "golden melt-in-the-mouth meat" and does it ever! It is a finely sliced pork fillet cooked so that it actually melts in your mouth.

The meal is not only marvelous, but our bill comes to under ten dollars U.S. We all want this chef to cook for us all the time. Everything about the place is comfortable and excellent. Even at this busy lunch time, the woman serving the food takes the time to write the names of the dishes in my notebook, so I will have them accurately in Chinese. Thanks to the generosity of strangers, I have had the best hole-in-the-wall food of my trip and one of the most memorable for the pleasure of good company.

I take some photos and then we walk past some markets selling crafts and household goods. I tag along to learn some local bargaining techniques. We say goodbye and I have some time before my next interview. They are surprised I am not only going alone but going without a translator.

I go to the Beijing Hotel for a taxi because I know someone there will give careful instructions to the driver. Even though I have the name and number written in Chinese and the route penned on the map, I have been told the Li Family Restaurant is hard to find. It is. My driver is very helpful and it is great to have him wait and make a round trip. We reach our destination circuitously through streets only seen in old black-and-white photographs of China in the twenties. We have stopped at a walled courtyard with the name Li painted on a board.

Mr. Li and his oldest daughter come to meet me. We go into a front room where a large table takes up most of the space. There is a plastic lazy susan in the middle of the table, red restaurant chairs around it, and a few more against the wall. There is a sink in one corner of the room and a coat rack in another. We sit down. On the back wall is a kite, an ordinary bird-like one, that often gets flown. On another wall are three characters in wonderfully brushed calligraphy that translate to Li Family Cuisine. It was done by Pu Jie, the brother of the last emperor, a calligrapher of national reputation.

Mr. Li's English is fine and he starts out by telling me that cooking is his hobby. He retired from teaching applied mathematics at the Beijing Economic Institute in 1990 at the age of 70. The restaurant was opened in 1985. He likes to cook with the tenderest pork fillet and with Mandarin fish, which he thinks is the best freshwater fish. A recipe for it that the Dowager Empress Cixi liked is prepared with ginger, garlic, scallions, and different herbs.

He also does a sweet-and-sour taste fish with green peppers, bamboo shoots, ginger, and *aiyuk*, a Chinese plant. He prefers the local vinegar, which is a light-brown color, though he cooks with Camel brand salad oil from Hong Kong, which he sometimes mixes with sesame oil and peanut oil. He uses mainly woks and regular pots to boil dumplings. In his small kitchen, steamers are rarely used. He makes wheat flour dumplings filled with vegetables, pork, shrimp, a bit of egg, minced scallions, ginger, and bamboo shoots. Occasionally he makes a special dumpling with tomato flavored with soy sauce. Sometimes he makes pumpkin dumplings for his family. He makes a fried turnip cake using shredded turnip mixed with white pepper, ginger, carrot, wheat flour, and a bit of salt. The cakes are then shaped and fried. To fry them he uses peanut oil blended with a little rapeseed oil and sesame oil. He also bakes little sesame buns that are split and eaten with spicy shredded pork. The soup he prefers to cook is a hearty chicken soup, made from free-range soup chickens. It is served to his guests with winter melon, coriander, and water lily slices.

For dessert he favors the traditional sugar-coated caramelized tiny red apples, called the king of fruit. He said this fruit is also called *hung guar* or red fruit, as well as *sha li hun* or *arshunja*. He told me about the little red berry called *gouqizi* (sometimes translated as wolfberry) that is grown in many courtyards and is used for tea. It may be left to stand in liquor to make it more beneficial. A drink he likes, called *haw nectar*, is a blend of *gouqizi*, honey, and carrots.

I ask Mr. Li how this restaurant came to be so famous all over the world and he said that in 1984 CCTV (China Central T.V.) and *China Food* magazine had a nation-wide family banquet competition to celebrate the thirty-fifth anniversary of the People's Central Government. There were 2,900 contenders. All the candidate families prepared a banquet. Li Li, the Li family second daughter, had graduated from China Social University with a degree in food nutrition. When she won first prize, many Chinese newspapers reported the news and the *China Daily* interviewed her. In 1985 she had the idea for opening the restaurant in the front room of their home. Reservations are now booked months in advance.

Four and one-half years ago she and her brother, who is a dentist, emigrated to Melbourne, Australia, and started a joint venture called Li Li's. In 1991 Mr. Li, his wife, and granddaughter traveled to Australia for the opening. The family has since traveled to Hong Kong and Singapore for several weeks each to represent China and prepare its court cuisine in each place.

When he doesn't eat his own food or that of other Chinese chefs, Mr. Li likes to eat simple broiled steak or pork chops and sometimes a Western-style stewed chicken. I ask him what his new hobby is now that his old hobby has become a famous profession. He said it is watching the news and sports on T.V.

Saturday

Early on this beautiful morning I meet the driver for the drive to the Great Wall (*Wanli Changcheng*). The wall was started in 7 B.C.E. and it is mainly the portion completed during the Ming Dynasty that is to be seen at Badaling.

Traffic is typically heavy, but as we get close the driver is speeding at one hundred kilometers per hour for the last twenty minutes. Signs start to appear in several languages. In English I read: "Our Yangchiang County welcomes you," "Great Wall Pet World," "Protecting Wild Life is Protecting Humans," "China North International Shooting Range," "Ming Dynasty Waxworks Palace," "Going Places Toilet," and "A More Open China is Waiting for You."

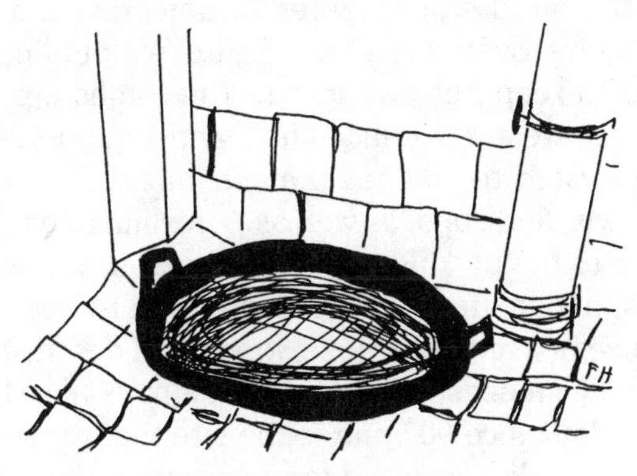

Wok over Fire-Hole in Tile Stove

We pass cars, vans, and buses on the road and can see watchtowers on the hills as we approach one of the seven wonders of the ancient world. This north pass was one of the Wall's most heavily secured gates because it safeguarded Beijing. The terrain is vast and mountainous. The closer we get we can see large tourist restaurants, food stalls, and vendors of every description. The parking lot, as might be expected, is enormous and is crowded, even at this early hour. On either side of the entry to the north gate are restaurants, refreshment stands, film and information centers, shopping areas, a philately center, a post office, and more.

Facts can be researched and pictures admired, but the keenness of apprehension cannot. The resonance of walking along with throngs of others, through the currents of strong winds, on the Great Wall of China, a place central to the history of civilization, is the kind of experience that keeps me from being an armchair traveler.

I meet the driver, who is eating with friends, and browse until they have finished. We are on our way to the Ming Tombs, which were built from 1409–1644 and are known in China as *Shisan Ling* ("The Thirteen Tombs") because thirteen of the sixteen Ming Dynasty emperors are buried there. I have not eaten since early morning, and I go to the crowded Ding Ling restaurant and order *dan dan mein*, which is served in a styrofoam container. I take it outside and sit on a bench watching the crowd. The noodles are hot and tasty, not pasty as I feared.

This is a necropolis of beauty and ritual with stone lions, serpents, dragons, and phoenixes. The largest stele in China is here, positioned on a tortoise, a symbol of longevity. There is a famous sacred road lined with paired stone figures of unicorns, camels, and elephants, and twelve oversized stone figures of public officials. The road is curved to keep out evil spirits. The tombs are intricate and each has a tortise stele, a sacrificial hall, and an underground palace. One of the excavated tombs has a museum that includes gold and jade plates, bowls, and cups, as well as porcelain ones.

The avenue to the parking lot is like a bazaar; vendors are selling expensive furs, paper kites, children's games, antique replicas, film, postcards, souvenirs, and, of course, food of all descriptions.

In the evening I meet some people at Beihai Park, which has been an imperial garden since 907 and is the site that Kublai Khan chose for his palace. Its lakes were added over centuries and during the

Ming Dynasty the famous White Dagoba was built on the site of the destroyed palace on Hortensia Island. The *dagoba* is a white Tibetan-styled *stupa* that was built in 1651 to honor the first Dalai Lama to visit Beijing. It was rebuilt in 1731 and is decorated with inscriptions and figures devoted to Buddha and Lamaist deities.

On my last evening in Beijing I am pleased to be part of a banquet arranged at the Fangshan Restaurant located in Beihai Park. It is housed in several imperial halls that last served the Dowager Empress Cixi. It is said that Cixi's favorite food were the small baked cornflour buns stuffed with spicy lamb that someone served on the side of the road when she was very hungry. Variations of this dish are still made and served in this restaurant that was established in 1925 by chefs from the court. The restaurant has been in these halls since 1956 and offers two hundred dishes from Chi'ing Dynasty menus.

The food is in the style of the royal households, and there are dishes that can be traced back to the Han Dynasty. Some are said to be the favorites of the Dowager Empress Cixi. The restaurant is a study in the history of Chinese cuisine as well as a terrific place for a dinner party.

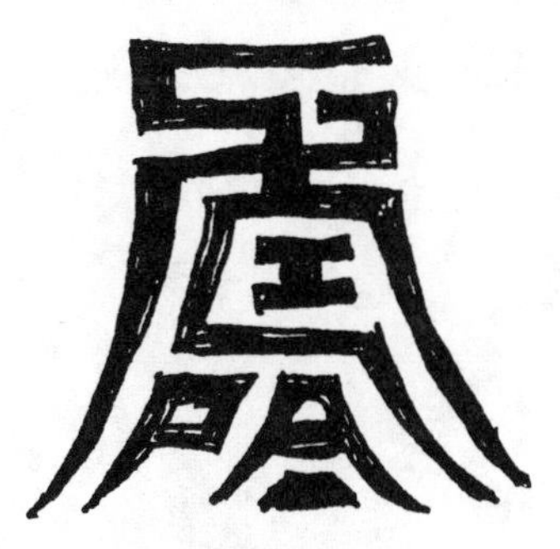

Symbol for Happiness

4

Shanghai and the East

The most populated city in the world is located on a delta in the East China Sea at the mouth of the Yangtse, the greatest river in Asia. Thousands of years ago it was a fishing village; in 751 C.E. it was still a fishing village. Shanghai means "on the sea." During the Sung Dynasty (960–1279 C.E.) it became known as *Shanghai Zhen* or "market town on the sea." Large ships can traverse the river to Sichuan and then head north on the Grand Canal, while smaller ships can visit hundreds of towns and villages. In summer rice is the prevailing crop and in winter, wheat and barley.

During the seventeenth century Shanghai became a port and by 1756 the British East India Company established trade there, mainly in woolen goods. In 1842, the British captured Shanghai, which then had a population of half a million. The Chinese paid the equivalent of a quarter of a million dollars to the British to fend off looting and destruction. The city was divided according to the Treaty of Nanking, in which the good news and the bad news were hard to tell apart. The city was not sacked and was opened to foreign trade; British, French, and eventually Japanese regions were established, each with their own legal and political systems. For years, Chinese insurgents living in a walled section of the city tried to no avail to stop the opium trade that outsiders were promulgating and to restore the Ming Dynasty.

Shanghai has since been the site of many uprisings. In 1915 there was a student-worker demonstration against the Japanese. In 1921 the first Communist Party Congress was held there. The British quashed a strike in 1925 and anti-imperialist activity in the city escalated. In 1927 Chiang Kaishek attacked the Communist Party, initiating what was regarded as a period of civil war that continued until the invasion of the Japanese in 1937. The revolutionary battles started up again as soon as the Japanese surrendered in 1945. On October 1, 1949 the People's Republic of China was proclaimed by Chairman Mao Zedong in Beijing.

Shanghai has always been a very international city. A city of commerce, agriculture, science, and industry, it is also a shopper's destination. People from all over China walk the streets of Shanghai window shopping and buying goods not available in such quality and quantity in many other parts of the country. The buildings along the Bund and other areas reflect European and Japanese architecture and design. Nanjing Road is a shopping street that runs from the Bund ("bund" is an Anglo-Indian word for an artificial embankment along a shore; in this case it is the Huangpu River's banks that are held back by bunding). It is said that the Shanghai #1 Department Store gets 100,000 customers a day.

Wednesday Evening

It is raining as the taxi crawls through rush-hour traffic to the Shanghai Sheraton Hotel. I will learn that it never takes less than an hour to get anywhere by car in Shanghai. Don't bother asking why because the response is always "*Mei you wen ti*," or "No problem!" We pass a large billboard that says in many languages: "Evergreen Golf and Country Club–36 holes with 36 kinds of moods."

I go to dinner with Joshua Gu and Tsang Kam Fai, chief of the Chinese kitchen. This turns out to be one of those rare meals you never forget. What is impressive is that we order from the menu of the twenty-sixth floor restaurant Guan Yue Tai (Palace for Appreciating the Moonlight). The only "usual" cold plates are the thinly sliced five-flavor beef and the marinated roast pork slices. In addition we have lovely textured jellyfish, *ba zao yu* (smoked squid), *hai cai* (seaweed), *hai yan*, tiny little dried fish soaked until chewy, and *shisamo* (translated as "capelin"), small fried sardines.

For starters we have squid in hot pepper sauce, the texture soft and creamy against the bite of the peppers. There are scallops sauteed with *gouqizi* (wolfberries), another innovative combination, and then *xin ren zhi zhu* and *dai yu* (hair-tail fish with ginkgo nuts, bean curd, and preserved vegetables). This is such a savory combination and though the little bones are annoying, it is worth the effort. Next is gluten, cooked and sauced to taste like duck liver. With this we sip Shaoxing wine. I am pleased that this time it was the chef who sent it back when it was served to me cold. It came back at the proper temperature in a small carafe placed in warm water.

We are waiting for the hairy crabs. The crabs are steamed and served with Chinkiang vinegar for dipping. My hosts are divided over which morsel to eat first; I follow the chef and start with the smallest claws then move to the front ones. I then turn the crab over, remove the tail, and break the carapace apart. The back is now a bowl filled with crabmeat, roe, and the steamed juices; add a little vinegar and it is delicious. This is clearly the best part. We use all our tools: a claw cracker, a double pick with one end curved like a buttonhook and the other straight, and a curved flat-bladed knife the size of a butter knife.

The sauce is Chinkiang vinegar with a bit of minced ginger and sugar. The tea served with it is a combination of ginger, black tea, and sugar. This is one of the rare occasions where Chinese tea is sweetened. After eating, finger bowls of tea and lemon slices freshen the hands and mouth. I describe Maryland crab feasts with their hammers and my companions say that at home they use little mallets as well. We talk about different kinds of crabs and where they can be found. The best quality of the green thin-shelled Shanghai hairy crab comes from Yang Zhou Lake. The she-crab is best eaten in October and the he-crab in November.

We talk about how pollution is destroying the oceans and ocean life. Here, too, they do not use many local scallops or clams because of the water conditions. There is a lot of seeding and aquaculture. I realize most travelers don't realize how aware good chefs are of food quality. We talk about conservation and progress; of nature, of cuisine, and of culture. I ask about some calligraphy that looks to be in a familiar style. I am told it is the last emperor's brother who did it. I say "Oh, Pu Jie," and the chef, surprised that I am at all in touch, asks to go on a food hunt with me on Friday, so I am pleased. It is almost 11:00 and the three of us, who sat down as strangers, have been eating and talking for almost three hours.

Thursday

I have a room-service breakfast and sort my notes. Later I meet with Paul Hoeps, an executive chef, and Xu Jie, a deputy executive chef who is a specialist in Shanghainese food and foodlore. We make a plan to meet on Saturday at 5:00 A.M. to go to large food markets. He has made delicious onion cakes for me; they are small and not greasy.

At 11:30 I meet with a Sheraton executive and some people from the Shanghai Municipal Tourism Administration. We are quite a foursome. Everyone but Mr. Mei has a notebook and pen out, busily making notes. We order; I have the steamed fish with ginger and vinegar, served with soup and rice. Joshua has a similar lunch. The guests of honor have American soup, tuna salad with hard-boiled eggs, and one a cheeseburger with french fries, the other a fried egg and cheese sandwich with french fries, "as a change from hamburger."

For dinner I meet an interesting American woman whose office is near the American Embassy, which is a compound beautifully gardened in the British Colonial manner. We eat down the road from the Embassy at a hole-in-the-wall place called Wei Gong or Abundant Palace. Neither part of the name seems to apply. I ask my acquaintance to order since this is her turf. Her Chinese is enviable; it sounds so authentic to my ears. The cadence of many Westerners, as even I can tell, is just a bit off.

We have *niurou ban*, thinly sliced beef cooked at the table on a preheated metal platter (an extremely old form of cooking in China) with red onions, garlic, green peppers, scallions, soy sauce, and some red peppers. We also try the *Mapo dofu* (hot spicy Sichuan style), *doumio* (peabean shoots—quite delicious and almost never used in the U.S.) and *yu xi'ang qie zi* (eggplant with fish fragrance), one of my "home style" favorites.

Friday

I leave the hotel early and go to Yu Yuan Garden. One of the most famous gardens in South China, it was built from 1559–1577. Its neighborhood, now called the Yu Yuan Market, seems to be the model for America's "Chinatowns." In 1858 this was the location of the secret "small sword society" that held much of the city under its control. The entrance to the garden is in the neighborhood's center, past streets of shops and alleys of stalls selling everything from pearls to sacks of balloons, from cashmere sweaters to fifty-cent aprons. Once inside there is a square within a square, and in the middle of the zig-zagged path across a small pond is the famous Wu Xing Ting teahouse, a wooden structure that has been there for several hundred years and has been depicted in art and poetry. I go in and am seated upstairs near a window. It is a little after eight and though the street and park are filling up, the teahouse is quiet. I have come after the regulars and before the tourists, so I am enjoying a rare moment of quiet and the pleasure of physical space, a rarity in this most populated city. I have *bi luo chuan*, green tea and a set collection of breakfast nibbles. This includes small pillows of *dofu*, tea eggs (made with quail eggs), flavored rice wrapped in a lotus leaf and tied with string, and *xien mei*, small green preserved plums that are delicious. As I leave, I am given a small souvenir book, a reproduction of the *Book of Tea*.

Walking across the path with nine bends that zig-zags the pond, I enter the now very crowded scholar's house and garden with its beautiful studies, intricate walkways, carp pools, rock gardens, and covered paths. These aspects of the house and garden have been in their present formation since 1560. I walk into a shop at the back and see some old ink stones and other writing material that seem good quality. I buy what is, of course, a reproduction of an old, slightly reddish inkstone with an "eye" in the stone near the carved dragon.

I walk out and wander a back alley so crowded there is no air space between pedestrians. It seems to be a dry-goods market with sewing threads, zippers, and buttons. There is cart after cart with similar arrays. I turn a corner and now the stalls offer "buy them by the dozen" plastic toys and trinkets. These are the convoluted alleyways in which, during their heyday, it would have been very foolish for a Western woman to browse alone.

I walk along the Bund where the architecture is surprisingly international. Many of its buildings were built in the twenties and thirties in the art deco and arts and crafts styles. I turn onto Nanjing Lu and take a look at the Peace Hotel, whose lobbies and dining and dance halls have seen more than their share of history. As I walk on this main shopping street, I am overwhelmed by the crowds in the stores.

Here one can buy modern consumer goods of every description and every price: arts and crafts, books and scrolls, as well as the "four treasures of study"—brushes, ink, ink stones, and paper.

I go on to another area; a large central market where, even though it is late in the day, the produce looks good and the fish in the tanks seem healthy. It is reassuring to see white-suited chefs shopping here. There are butcher stalls as well as areas for cold cuts, sausages, and dried chicken. Ready-to-cook prepared but raw dishes are being sold. This is a popular form of convenience shopping, since all the ingredients don't have to be purchased separately. I am told that whatever isn't eaten for dinner will be eaten for breakfast. An old New York Chinese food habit turns out to be authentic. At a cooked food stall across from the market, I buy a small rolled *dofu* skin savory and a few pieces of fried and seasoned wheat gluten. Both are quite good. The array of packaged food at a nearby supermarket attests to the popularity of both canned and frozen food.

I get back to the hotel and am ready for an early dinner at the Guan Yue Tai Restaurant. The restaurant has been featuring an extraordinary specialty; Tsang Kam Fai, one of the best and most knowledgeable chefs I have ever encountered, has designed a dinner that is described in Chapter 9. I enjoy it as we eat to the accompaniment of Chinese classical music supplied by the quartet of Zeng, Pipa, Erh Hu, and Yang Qing.

Saturday

In the morning at 5:50 A.M. I meet Xu Jie for what he calls the best street breakfast in China. We go to Wu Ding Lu, a cross-section of a street market.

First we have *xin jin bao*, doughy *jiaozi* stuffed with ground pork leg and some of its skin, the juice of ground scallions mixed with sesame oil, minced ginger, and some Haio soy sauce. Before they are cooked the dumplings are sprinkled with black sesame seeds. In a *wok* over a wood fire, these dumplings are put into a mixture of oil and water. They are covered and cooked for fifteen minutes, then the cover is removed and the bottoms of the dumplings are browned until crisp. These are served really hot. The secret to eating them is first to nibble a little hole and suck out the juice (being careful not to burn yourself). They are eaten with vinegar. You know they are good (and cheap) because this is the first place I have seen so many young children eating.

Next we have what is described to me as real *wonton* soup in a porkbone stock. I am quickly informed that there is no MSG in any of this and that up until twenty years ago it was never used and is now being dropped again as people learn more about it. The soup's stock is enhanced with herbs (greens) and white pepper. Xu Jie says the white pepper used in this area in the food ensures that there is no need for msg. The *wonton* are the texture you hope for: really soft without falling apart and very distinctive in the delicious broth. This would bring *wonton* soup back to fancy restaurants.

The next course is a slice of fried rice loaf. It is really crunchy on the outside and creamy in the middle, made, I am told, from three kinds of rice. Next we share a street breakfast bestseller: a *you tiao* (an oil stick—a long, twisted unsweetened cruller, often eaten with soy milk) wrapped in a *shaobing*, in this case, a yeast wheat-dough bread baked with sesame seeds and scallions. My host tells me he knows people from "the white nations" would like this food.

He also tells me that in Xi'an one of the reasons cumin is used is to keep food moist, because the emperor of the Chi'ing found the wood fires made the food too dry. He explains that it is a shame I can-

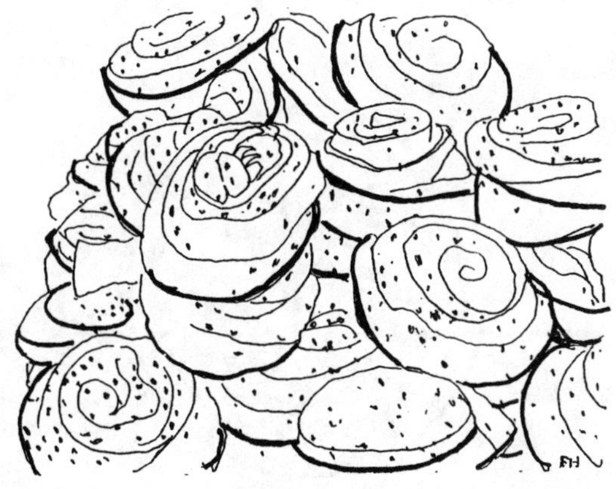

Sesame Seed Buns

not get to Wuxi and I tell him I would very much have liked to. He says that in many places they still cook over straw there and it gives the rice a special taste.

We go through the farmer's market where people come to sell fruit, vegetables, grains, and beans in great variety. We nibble on some raisins from Xinjian 1,800 miles away.

It is now 7:00 A.M. and we go back to the hotel. I pack and then go to the metal goods store for some cleavers and food preparation tools. The clerks are very patient with me, though the store is crowded. I make my selections and then notice a comedy of manners. After I collect what I came for, I look at what other people are buying and try to learn. Then I notice some are buying what I have just bought. I can tell from their dress that many are from restaurants and hotels and won't be out of pocket, but I worry anyway. The cleavers I know are reported to be the best and the deep dragon and phoenix cutters also, but as for the rest . . . .

My lunch appointment is the first no-show I have had. This exception makes me realize how well my schedule has been going. I have little time before my flight, so I go to the "deli" and order a curried chicken salad that arrives so filled with mayonnaise it is inedible. I order some vegetarian sushi that is delicious, and it encourages me to try a bit of chestnut cake. The European pastry influence in Shanghai is visible everywhere. The Western influence on bread, cake, and other pastries is white flour and sugar. The cakes look as opulent and taste as decadent as they do everywhere.

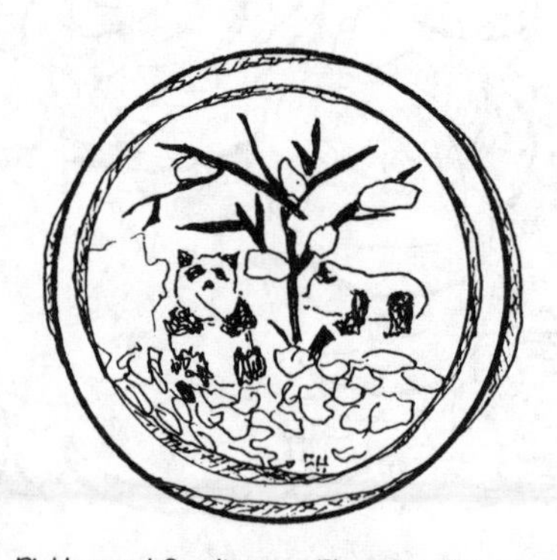

Pickles and Condiments Plated as Pandas

I am seen to a taxi by Joshua Gu, who has his notes for me, in English. He and Chef Tsang have been my teachers in Shanghai, and are much appreciated.

In general, central Chinese cooking is lighter, uses less oil, has more sweetness, and is presented on individual plates more often than in other parts of China. There are some international surprises as well because Shanghai has been a destination and residence for foreigners for hundreds of years. Even borscht is ubiquitous here.

One can find dishes from Kiangsi, called the "Land of Fish and Rice" (as in the "Land of Milk and Honey"). Chekiang dishes are served as well, one example being *hsia pa*, fish-head stew with wine and vinegar, brown sauce, and rice. Tea-smoked pomfret, fish smoked over black tea leaves in a *wok* for half an hour, and pan-fried carp with rice-wine cakes and bamboo shoots are popular dishes.

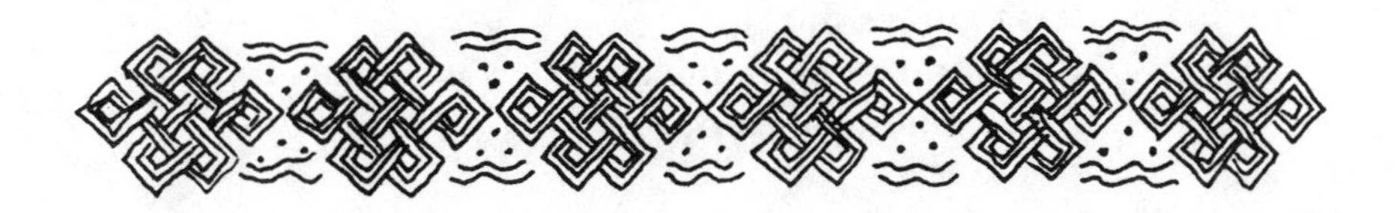

Drunken Chicken Tsui Chi

1	5 lb.	roasting chicken
1	T.	coarse salt
1	T.	granulated sugar
2	C.	Shaoxing rice wine (dry sherry may be substituted)
1		small bunch Chinese parsley (cilantro) for garnish (Italian flat-leafed parsley may be substituted)

Rub chicken inside and out with salt and sugar mixture. Refrigerate 1 hour. With cleaver remove wings and drumsticks and cut the carcass in half lengthwise. Then cut each half across into 4 pieces. Place the chicken in a bowl and cover with 1 cup of the wine. Marinate 6 hours or overnight.

Heat steamer and place the chicken in the steamer for 45 to 60 minutes until fully cooked, but not overcooked. Remove the chicken and place it in a bowl with 1 cup of the wine. Cover and refrigerate for 24 hours. If you are going to wait longer than 24 hours before serving, discard the wine and cover the chicken until ready to serve. Serve garnished with parsley. *8 servings*

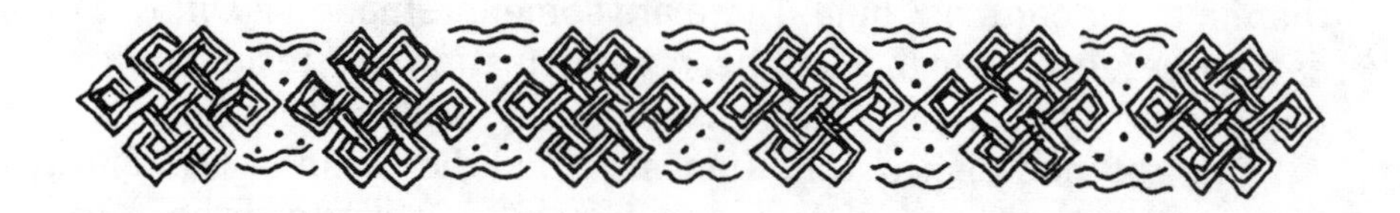

Shanghai Lion's Head (Yangzhu See Jee Too) (Cantonese)

1	lb.	coarsely ground pork
1	t.	fresh ginger, minced
1	t.	dried orange peel, minced
1	T.	green onion, minced
1	t.	soy sauce
1	T.	Shaoxing wine (dry sherry may be substituted)
1	t.	sugar
1	T.	cornstarch
1		egg white, beaten
1/4	t.	salt
1/4	t.	white pepper

Broth

4	C.	chicken stock
1	t.	minced ginger
3	T.	soy sauce
1	t.	sugar
1 1/2	lb.	Chinese cabbage (preferably Shanghai bok choi)
8		dried Chinese mushrooms, soaked in hot water for 20 minutes and drained

To make the meatballs (lion's heads), mix pork, ginger, orange peel, green onion, soy sauce, Shaoxing, sugar, cornstarch, egg white, salt, and white pepper. Form into 8 meatballs and set aside.

In a clay pot with cover or other flame-proof pot, heat the broth and add ginger, soy sauce, and sugar. Shred cabbage, add to the pot, and bring to a boil. Add mushrooms. Lower heat under broth until it is simmering. Carefully add meatballs and simmer for an hour. *8 servings*

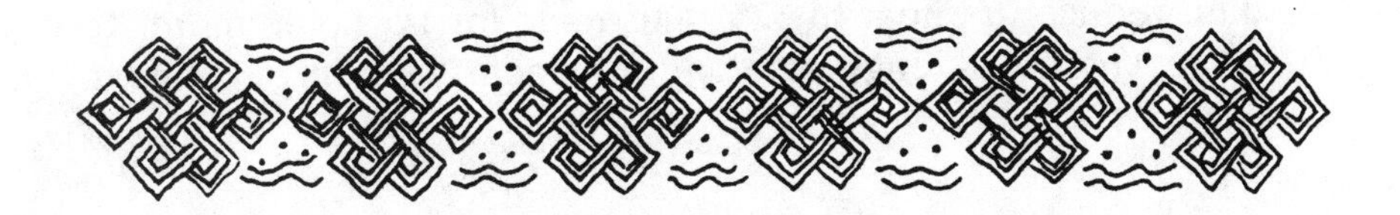

Eight Treasure Shanghai Duck

1		boned duck (5–6 lb.)
1	T.	coarse salt
1	C.	glutinous rice
½	C.	long-grain rice
2		Chinese duck liver sausages (other Chinese sausages may be substituted)
3	T.	peanut oil (safflower oil may be substituted)
8		Chinese dried black mushrooms, soaked in hot water for ½ hour and diced
12		chestnuts, boiled or roasted, then peeled and sliced
8		fresh water chestnuts, peeled and sliced
¼	C.	ginkgo nuts
2	3-inch	bamboo shoots, diced
2	T.	scallions, minced
2	T.	Chinese parsley, minced
1	t.	fresh peeled ginger, minced
¼	C.	Shaoxing rice wine (dry sherry may be substituted)
2	T.	soy sauce

Rinse duck, pat dry, and rub cavity with salt. Cook each type of rice according to directions. Cool the rice and stir together in a large bowl. Finely slice the sausages and stir into the rice blend. Preheat oven to 400°.

Heat oil in a *wok* or skillet on medium heat and stir fry all other ingredients except the wine and soy sauce for about 5 minutes. Mix the stir fry into the rice mixture with the wine and soy sauce. When cool enough to handle, stuff all duck cavities with mixture. Using a kitchen needle and thread or trussing skewers, close the openings. Set the duck on a rack in a roasting pan filled with an inch of water. Roast for 45 minutes at 400°, then reduce the heat to 325° and roast for 1¼ hours more. To serve, cut in half lengthwise and then across in four sections to make 8 pieces. *8 servings*

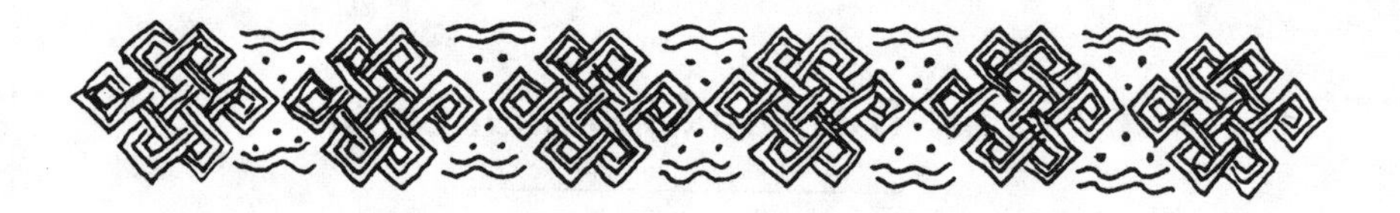

Sweet Red-Bean-Paste Pancakes (Tou Sha Kuo Bing)

2	eggs
½ t.	vanilla (optional)
½ C.	"instant" flour (all-purpose flour may be substituted)
¼ C.	cornstarch
1 C.	water
6 oz.	sweet red-bean paste
¼ C.	peanut oil (safflower oil may be substituted)

Mix the eggs, vanilla, flour, cornstarch, and water and stir so that there are no lumps. In a small bowl mix the red-bean paste so that it is spreadable. Pour the oil into an 8-inch skillet and heat. Pour off the excess oil and reserve. Pour in half the batter and tilt the pan so that it flows evenly to make an 8-inch pancake. Working quickly, spread half the bean paste on half the pancake with a heatproof rubber spatula. Fold the pancake in half and seal the edges. Remove from the heat and repeat the procedure with the second half of the batter and filling. Cut each pancake into four small wedges and serve hot. These may be made before dinner and heated, crisped in oil, and sliced just before serving.

8 servings

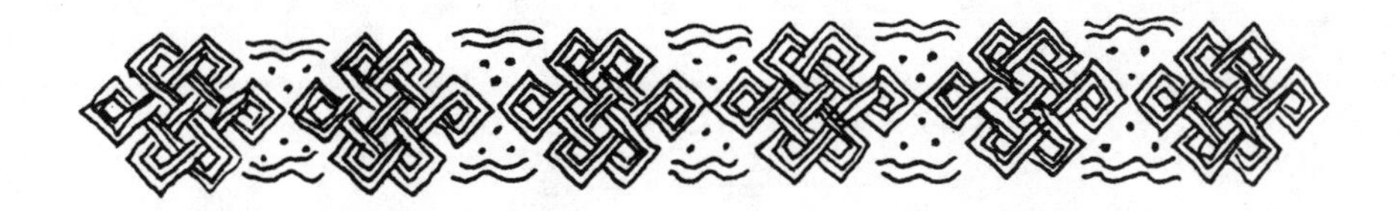

Hair-Tail Fish with Salted Vegetables

4	oz.	salted vegetables (*chao zhou*)
2	oz.	ginkgo nuts
2	oz.	dried bean curd rolls
1	lb.	hair-tail fish
1/4	lb.	fresh white mushrooms, sliced
1	oz.	fresh ginger, sliced
1	bunch	spring onions, sliced
2	medium	carrots, sliced
1	medium	leek, rinsed well and sliced
1	T.	sugar
1	C.	chicken stock
1	t.	white pepper
1	t.	fish sauce

Put salted vegetables, ginkgo nuts, and dried bean curd rolls in boiling water for 5 minutes, then remove, drain, and slice. Cut the hair-tail fish into bite-sized pieces and deep fry for 6 minutes. Remove the fish from the oil. Place 2 tablespoons of oil in the *wok*, heat, and add mushrooms, ginger, spring onions, carrots, and leek, and stir fry for 5 minutes. Add sugar, pepper, fish sauce, salted vegetables, ginkgo nuts, dried bean curd, and hair-tail fish. Stir fry for 3 minutes while adding chicken stock.

4 servings

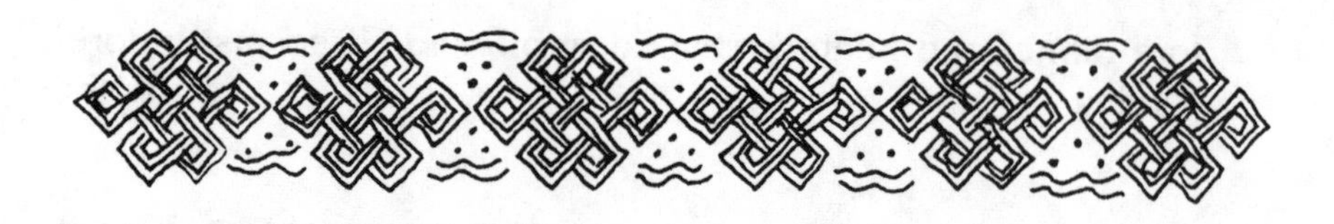

Sauteed Scallops with Wolfberry

1	lb.	small scallops
1	T.	cornstarch
1	t.	fresh ginger, minced
1	t.	fresh garlic, minced
1	T.	scallions, minced
2	oz.	(*gouqizi*) wolfberries, soaked and drained
1		pinch of salt
1/4	t.	white pepper
1	t.	sugar
2	T.	peanut oil (safflower oil may be substituted)
3/4	C.	water

Toss the scallops in the cornstarch, then cook them in boiling water until done (3–4 minutes). Drain and set aside. Place oil in a *wok*, heat, and add scallops and all other ingredients. Saute briefly. Serve with rice.

6 servings

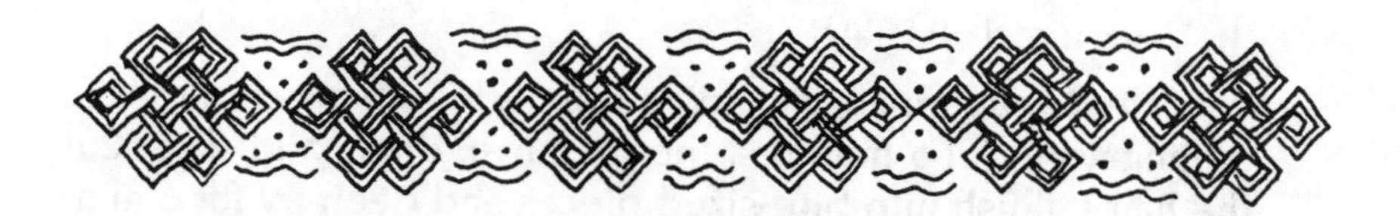

Sliced Cuttlefish with Chinese Brandy Sauce

1/2 lb.	cuttlefish (squid), sliced
1 oz.	XO or fish sauce (available in Chinese specialty stores)
1-inch piece	fresh ginger, peeled and minced
3 cloves	garlic, peeled and minced

1	pinch of salt
½ C.	chicken stock
⅓ t.	sugar
½ t.	cornstarch mixed with 2 T. of water

Slice the cuttlefish (squid) and poach in boiling water until cooked. Remove from water and drain. Heat oil in a *wok*. Add ginger, garlic, and XO or fish sauce. Stir fry for 1 minute, then add cuttlefish, stir, and add remaining ingredients. Serve with Chinese brandy sauce.

2 servings

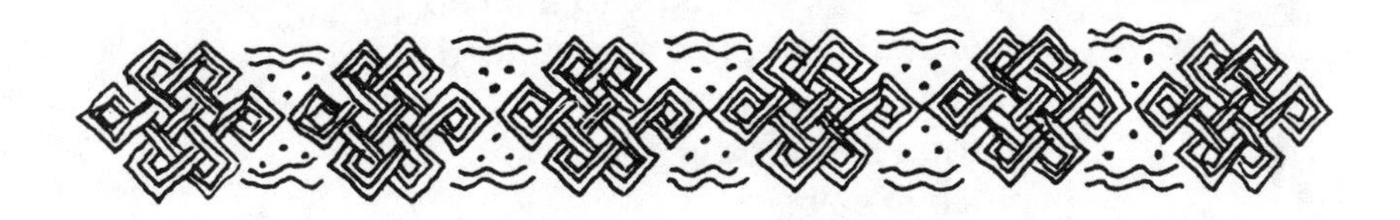

Chinese Brandy Sauce

2 oz.	Chinese chili paste
½ oz.	*conpoy* (dried scallops)
½ oz.	small dried shrimp
½ oz.	Jin Hua ham (Virginia ham may be substituted)
4	spring onions, minced
½-inch piece	ginger, peeled and minced
2 oz.	sesame oil
2 T.	Chinese brandy (cognac may be substituted)

Soak the *conpoy* and shrimp separately in hot water for 20 minutes, then drain and dice. Heat oil in a *wok*, add all other ingredients, and stir until well amalgamated.

2 servings

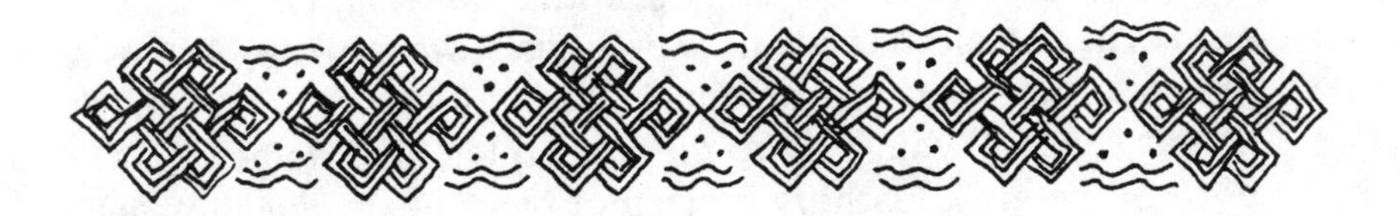

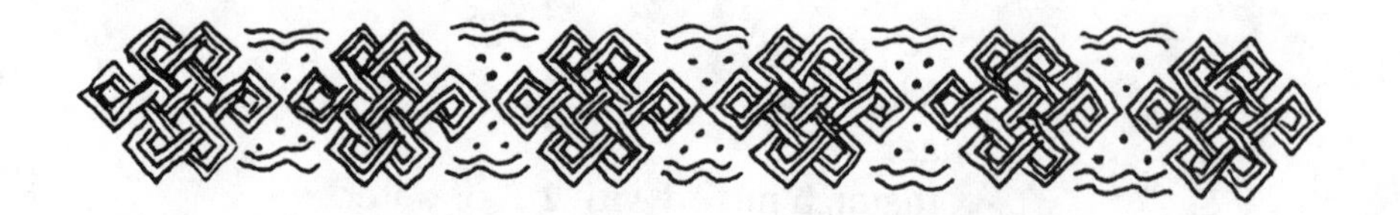

Diced Gluten with Oyster Sauce

$^3/_4$ lb. cooked gluten rolls or pieces (*main jin*)
2 T. ground chili pepper
1 oz. fresh ginger, peeled and minced
4 cloves fresh garlic, peeled and minced
1 T. plus 1 t. rock sugar
2 T. bottled oyster sauce
1 pinch of salt
$^1/_2$ C. chicken stock

Cut gluten into bite-sized pieces and deep fry. Remove and drain. Heat a small amount of oil in a *wok* add all ingredients except the gluten and stock. Stir until well amalgamated, then add stock and fried gluten. Serve immediately. *4 servings*

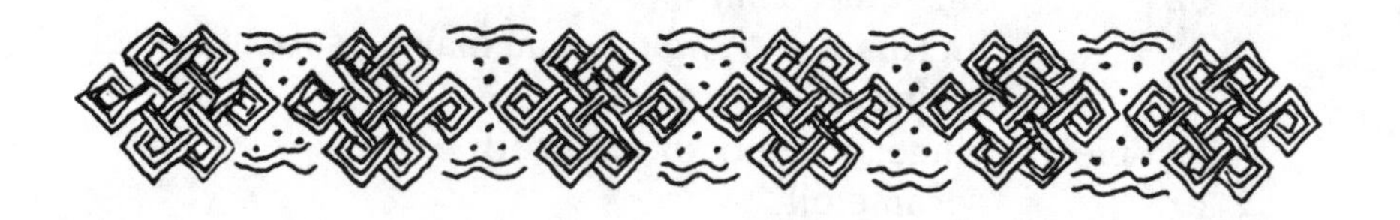

Shanghai Hairy Crab (Mo Hai)

How to Eat

The male has an oval breastplate with a bell-shaped circumference. The female has a full oval-shaped breastplate. First eat the small legs and pincer joints. Placing the crab on its back head away from you, pull up the breastplate and detach it. Dispose of the grey, feathery lungs and black heart. Eat the claws last. Serve with ginger tea, a finger bowl, and lemon.

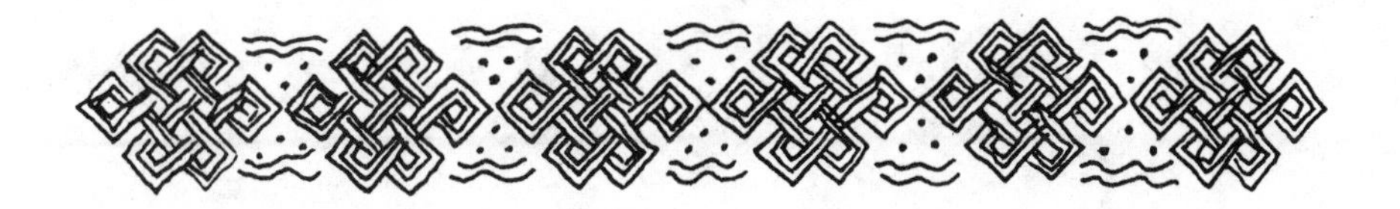

Shanghai Eel and Garlic (Chow Sin Wu)

1	lb.	eel, cleaned and filleted
1/4	C.	peanut or safflower oil
2	t.	fresh ginger, minced
2	cloves	garlic, minced
4		spring onions, chopped
12	cloves	garlic, peeled and sliced
1/2	lb.	bamboo shoots, sliced
1/2	C.	water
2	T.	light soy sauce
1/4	t.	finely ground white pepper
1	t.	sugar
1	t.	cornstarch dissolved in 1 T. cold water
1	T.	sesame oil
2	T.	Chinkiang vinegar

Blanch eel in boiling water, rinse under cold water, and drain. Cut into pieces about 1 inch by 2 inch. Heat oil in a *wok* and add the minced ginger, garlic, and scallions. When aromatic and lightly browned, add the eel and sliced garlic cloves. Lower the heat to medium and cook for 7 minutes. Add bamboo shoots and stir. Mix together water, soy sauce, pepper, sugar, and cornstarch. Pour the mixture over the eel, raise the heat and stir until well blended. Place the eel on a warm platter. Put sesame oil and vinegar into the hot *wok* and then pour over the eel. Serve immediately. *6 servings*

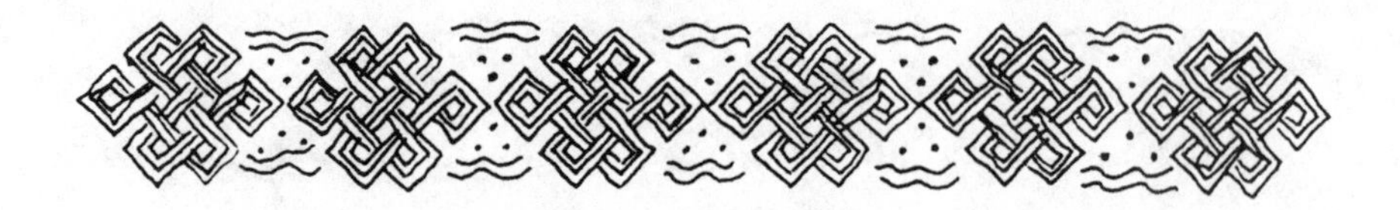

Chicken Fried in Walnuts (T'ao Jen Chi Ting)

1	lb.	boneless chicken thighs, skin removed
1		egg white
1	T.	cornstarch dissolved in 2 T. water
1	T.	soy sauce
1	C.	shelled walnuts
2	T.	peanut or safflower oil
12		paper-thin slices of fresh ginger
4		spring onions
1		green bell pepper
1		red bell pepper
2	T.	soy sauce
2	T.	Shaoxing rice wine or dry sherry
2	t.	brown sugar
		oil for deep frying (approximately 4 C.)

Cut the chicken into walnut-sized pieces. Mix together the lightly beaten egg white with 1 T. of the soy sauce and the cornstarch mixture. Marinate the chicken in this mixture for 20–30 minutes. Brown the walnuts in a 350° oven, then crush like coarse meal and set aside. Dredge the marinated chicken in the walnuts and deep fry for about 1 minute. Slice the onions and the red and green peppers into 2-inch pieces and set aside with the sliced ginger. If the *wok* has been used for deep frying, pour the oil out and put 2 tablespoons of peanut or other oil in the *wok*. Stir fry the ginger, peppers, and spring onions, then add the remaining soy sauce, wine, and sugar. Place the mixture on a warm plate and top with the fried chicken. Serve immediately.

6 servings

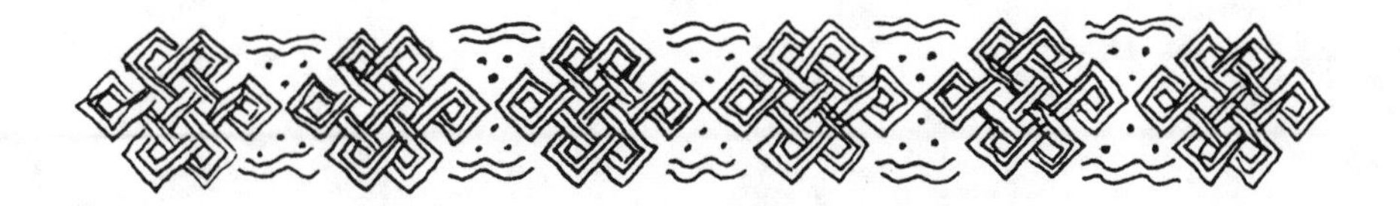

Sweet-and-Sour Fish Fillet (Sung Shu Huang Yu)

1½	lb.	firm white fish fillets, such as sea bass
1		whole egg
1		egg white
4	T.	flour
2	T.	cornstarch dissolved in 4 T. cold water
2	t.	rice vinegar
4–6	C.	oil for deep frying
½	C.	water
¼	C.	brown sugar
¼	C.	Chinkiang vinegar
¼	C.	commercial tomato ketchup
2	T.	soy sauce
1	t.	sesame oil
		Leaf lettuce in season, rinsed, dried, and with the leaves separated
		watercress for garnish

Cut the fish into 1½-inch squares. Prepare the batter by lightly beating the egg and the egg white with the flour, cornstarch mixture, and rice vinegar. Dip the fish in the batter and fry in hot oil for about 2 minutes. (The Western measure for temperature works if you are not using an automatic fryer. Drop a 1-inch cube of bread in hot oil. If it sinks to the bottom and comes to the surface within 2–4 seconds the oil is about 350°, the right temperature for deep frying most small morsels.) In a small heavy saucepan heat the water, sugar, Chinkiang vinegar, ketchup, soy sauce, and oil to create a sauce. Arrange the lettuce leaves on a warm platter, place the drained and blotted fish on the lettuce, pour the sauce over it, garnish with watercress, and serve immediately. *6 servings*

5

SICHUAN, HUNAN, GUILIN, AND THE WEST

My notes read, "Guilin—*Beauty*!" With a population of under a million, this 2,000-year-old city has been known as Guilin since the Ch'in Dynasty (221–207 B.C.). Guilin translates roughly as "cassia forest;" it was named for its cinnamon trees, since Shen Nung in 2700 B.C. discovered the uses of cinnamon and named the spice *kwei*, or, in *pinyin*, *gui*. This valuable spice has been the cause of many political and economic negotiations across millennia, since it has been favored by societies as diverse in time and culture as early Rome, medieval Italy, and present-day England. Guilin is one of the twenty-four cities protected by the government for their historical value.

My room at the Sheraton Guilin has a balcony and a view of the river and mountains. I am grateful and realize how I have longed for a landscape.

I have a light meal at the Guilin Food Court and then set out for a walk. Along the river is a bazaar where at dark vendors set up stalls lit with primus lanterns. The row along the river sells, in stall after stall, identical goods: tablecloths, pajamas, silk shirts, kimonos, and T shirts; all are of tourist quality. The street row is only slightly more varied; it also includes beads and "jade" antiques, undoubtedly made at the local "Antique Factory."

Sunday

After room service delivers delicious *congee*, fruit, and tea, which I eat on my balcony, I go to meet some people from the hotel's management staff who have arranged an outing. We take a van to a boat that looks like a version of the African Queen and are seated in a top deck cabin. We pull out and immediately I am in heaven; the boat engine is quiet and, except for absurdly loud blasts of the horn, we set off calmly down the river. My hosts have packed a lunch from the hotel, and once again I am enjoying food and comfortably sharing an adventure with strangers.

Guilin has been extolled in poetry and painting for its extraordinary scenery and a climate that permits this landscape to be explored and enjoyed. Geologists say that until the land thrust up 200 million years ago, the area was ocean. Its layers of limestone were carved by wind and water into the uniquely formed fingers of hills. Graceful mounds, peaks, caves, and underground streams line the banks of the Li River (a branch of the Pearl River). The six-hour ride from Guilin to Yangshou is like a dream as the boat glides through an ageless landscape reflected in the water. People still fish with cormorants from bamboo rafts. Tiered rice paddies and water buffalo complete the picture-perfect view. Over the years people have seen images in the mountains and cave formations, including camels, dragons, horses, elephants, and human vignettes. The stalactites and stalagmites are often enormous and varicolored. One can wander from downtown Guilin through hills and into caves the size of stadiums. Some caves have carved poems and sculpture; others have ancient graffiti. A Tang poet wrote:

> Weather in the Wuling ridges is hot.
> Only Guilin makes people feel pleasant.
> The rivers are like blue gauze belts,
> The mountains erect as kingfisher jade hairpins.

We get off the boat in Yangshou, a small town filled with trinket and souvenir stalls as well as hardware and stationery stores and language schools. The food is a mixture of local dishes and tourist inventions. Some of the restaurants are named in English: "Minnie Mao's," "Merry Planet Language Club," and "William's Barbecue." I realize I have not seen anything this kitschy in English since I have been here. We board a bus for the trip back to Guilin and the road takes us through farmland with vegetables, chickens, grain, and a very large brick factory. The brick are the wonderful red that is seen throughout this region and in many others.

Monday

I am in my room with the terrace door open and see the mountains and the river as well as the activity on the street. I am content and lazy, but decide to dress and walk to one of the large markets across the bridge and near Seven Star Park. The park is phenomenal and has one cave that is a mile long and filled with brilliant rock formations. One could easily spend a day exploring the park and its neighborhood.

With a cuisine very similar to that of Sichuan, further west, this area is one of the largest producers of processed chili peppers, in both dried and paste forms. In the markets, sacks and sacks are processed daily by large numbers of vendors. The region is rich in herbs, fish, produce, star anise, and, of course, cinnamon everywhere. Rice, sweet potatoes, sugar cane, grapefruit and other citrus fruit, water chestnuts, and taro fill the markets along with chestnuts, pears, and apples.

It is also a place that still sells the odd assortment of local game that includes civet, small deer, snakes, and almost unidentifiable small animals. I will say that this is off-putting to see; although it is a reasonable offering for a local market. Game dishes such as wild boar with fermented bean curd, river deer with bamboo shoots in brown sauce, and stewed turtle appear on some menus.

At 11:00 I meet with Stewart Wee, executive chef of the Guilin Sheraton, who is from Singapore, and Li Siu Chor, the Chinese executive chef. We talk about regional cuisine, and how Guilin cooking is a blend of Cantonese, Sichuan, and Northern cuisines, apart from the Guilin *mei fan* and the fact that people traditionally have eaten everything from rats to cats in this region. It is a rice-eating area and even the noodles are made from rice.

Pickles are a favorite; they are made from long beans, white radish, cabbage, peppers, and beans. The local Li River fish and produce such as cabbage, broccoli, cauliflower, French beans, Chinese cabbage, and bean sprouts certainly drive the cuisine. Pork, beef, quail, duck, and chicken are local. Cooks here use an Apollo oven to roast the duck and pork, which is suspended vertically. The cold dishes are boiled, including ingredients such as thinly sliced pork trotter, jellyfish, squid, sliced suckling pig, barbecued duck and pork, thinly sliced boiled beef (with other than the traditional five-flavor seasoning) and sliced chicken poached in soy sauce and water. Some of the dips for these include, vinegar, a local kind of tomato ketchup, garlic minced in vinegar, and, for the barbecue, a sauce with a base of sweetened preserved bean paste.

We talk about the markets, especially the number of people working with red pepper and garlic. Chef Wee praises the local mushrooms, both dried and fresh, and the fungi, and says he will make a lunch using local products.

I meet some people for lunch at the ground-floor Cathay Chinese Restaurant. To keep lunch light, we omit the cold course and start with a Guilin-style hot-and-sour soup, the difference being the use of *dofu* and local pickles for texture and flavor. It is really good. The Li River fish is a long, large-mouthed fish, steamed and tender. It looks like the drawings on the Benpo pottery. The fish is steamed, sprinkled with a julienne of ginger and spring onions which have been sauteed in a little oil, soy sauce, and local rice wine ("Three Flowers"). It is served whole and topped with sprigs of Chinese parsley. The beef dish is fillet sliced and marinated, then tossed with a bit of cornstarch, bicarbonate of soda, and finely ground white pepper. It is best marinated for at least six hours, then cooked and served hot with steamed broccoli. Guilin fried rice has some surprises: bits of pickle and dried fish. The fish is not odorous and just heightens the blandness of the rest of the mixture. We have a taste of spare ribs, which are sweet and hot. Dessert is a surprise—a scoop of banana ice cream and one of taro. Both are quite delicious and we talk about incorporating some Western techniques with Eastern ingredients. I tell them about my pomegranate and persimmon sorbets. They like the idea and will try it. The fresh fruit platter arrives and I can't even make a polite stab at it. It has been not only a good lunch, but an interesting hour.

I take my camera and go walking towards the street food and markets, thinking I will never eat again. But then I have to buy banana waffles; they are so great looking, I actually take a couple of bites. Why don't we have these as street food here? The stalls offer a lot of *mei fan*, steamed dumplings, dried fruit, candies, chestnuts, and melon seeds. I walk for three hours and then head back to the hotel. In the evening I go to a local concert.

Tuesday

I get up early and walk through the town to Elephant Trunk Hill. I am hungry but determined to have street food rather than eat in a restaurant. Finally, I find a vendor selling fried rice-flour cakes to a small crowd. One type of cake is filled with banana and the other with lotus paste. He also sells steamed, fried *wonton*.

Back at the hotel I arrange to go to the Buddhist Temple Restaurant that I saw Monday morning with the tour guide. For lunch I arrange to have a taxi take me to Xishan Hu Park. It is the location of the Ying Shi Liu Dong Miao (Buddhist temple). It is a small and serene temple and is maintained by monks who pray and study. They also run two restaurants; the larger one serves traditional food, but past the temple and up the hill is the Li Sa Chan Ting, a Buddhist restaurant. It is very empty, but the driver and I are greeted warmly. I start to leave, not wanting them to fuss for so few people, but they insist we sit down and bring tea immediately. I ask the driver to tell them to please bring a small amount of whatever they have already prepared. The tea is a good strong oolong, and soon a bowl of egg drop soup is set down in front of me. The broth is rich and flavorful and the texture of the egg drop is just the way it should be. The vegetable dish is a wrinkled squash, thinly sliced, and then absolutely creamy *dofu*, freshly made, served with a light ginger sauce. The rice is a local kind, with all sorts of vegetarian tidbits in it. It is a really wonderful and pleasant spot.

We leave there and go to the Li Jun Road and the Neng Ren Temple, which has an eating hall. I walk around the temple and am struck by the vivid personalities of its different rooms with their deities and altars and by the powerful effect each persona has. At an altar towards the end of the square I see what must be the Buddha that scares the hell out of you. With many heads and arms, it garishly assaults you with no apology. It is not one that I have seen in Mahayana or Zen Buddhism. I am pleased to be here, as it is clearly a center of activity. We are offered food but feel it would be gluttonous to accept.

Sichuan

Famous since the Han Dynasty for spicy and flavorful dishes, the richly endowed area of Sichuan has produced food for more than a thousand years that we would still recognize and enjoy today. In fact, although Sichuan seems a discrete culinary area, it has been, along with Hunan, more a source of tradition than a regional cuisine eaten only within a narrow geographical perimeter. Often called the "Brocade City" because of the exquisiteness of its weaving, Chengdu is the 2000-year-old provincial capital of Sichuan.

All over China, and indeed all over the world, various combinations of Sichuan brown "flower pepper" (*fagara*), chili peppers, fennel seed, coriander, sesame paste, vinegar, ginger, garlic, scallions, wine, and soy sauce are savored. Mao Zedong, who was from Hunan, is said to have had hot pepper incorporated into his bread. Steamed or fried

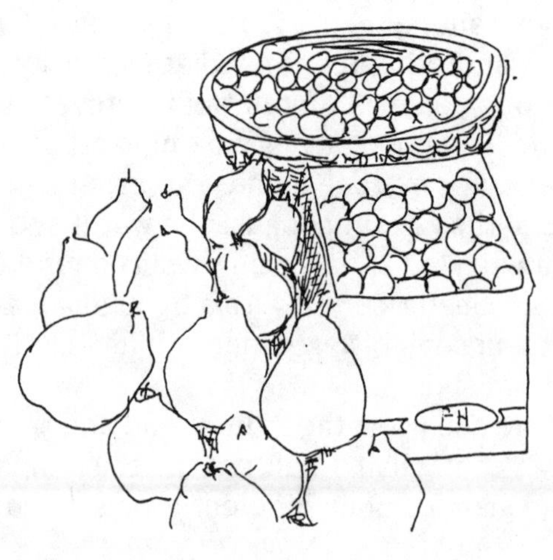

Pears and Chestnuts

bread and noodles are served more frequently in this region. The food of Hunan is similar, but sweet-and-sour sauce and steamed dishes are popular there as well.

In Sichuan vendors carry goods in bamboo buckets suspended from shoulder poles. China has always had a tradition of "take out," and these *dan dan* noodles have always been on the menu.

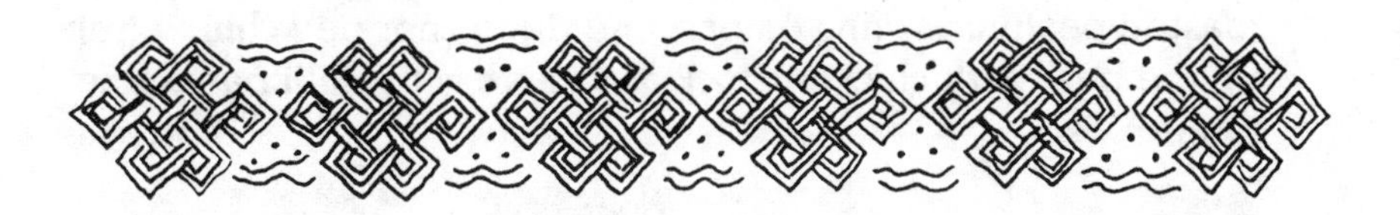

Guilin Rice Noodle (Courtesy of Li Siu Chor, Executive Chef, Guilin Sheraton)

400	g.	Guilin rice noodles, cooked
80	g.	beef shank
80	g.	pork belly with skin
1	pc.	anise
1	pc.	cassia bark
10	g.	ginger
1	pc.	bay leaf
10	g.	fermented soy beans
2	g.	nutmeg
20	ml.	soy sauce
200	ml.	water
5	g.	salt
10	g.	honey
80	g.	roasted peanuts
50	g.	spring onions
10	g.	dried whole chilies, chopped
400	ml.	chicken stock
		chili paste (optional)
		oil for deep frying

Make the sauce by mixing anise, cassia bark, ginger, bay leaf, fermented soy bean, nutmeg, soy sauce, and water and pour over the beef and boil for about 45 minutes, until fragrant. Add salt and honey to season. Remove beef and slice into strips and allow to cool. Boil pork in some salted water until cooked. Slice into strips and allow to cool. Re-heat noodles in boiling water and place in four bowls. Pour some of the fragrant sauce over the noodles. Heat some oil in a *wok* and deep fry the beef and the pork until crispy, place on top of the noodles. Sprinkle with roasted peanuts, spring onions, and dried chopped chilies. Top up the bowl with chicken stock and serve with chilli paste if required.

4 servings

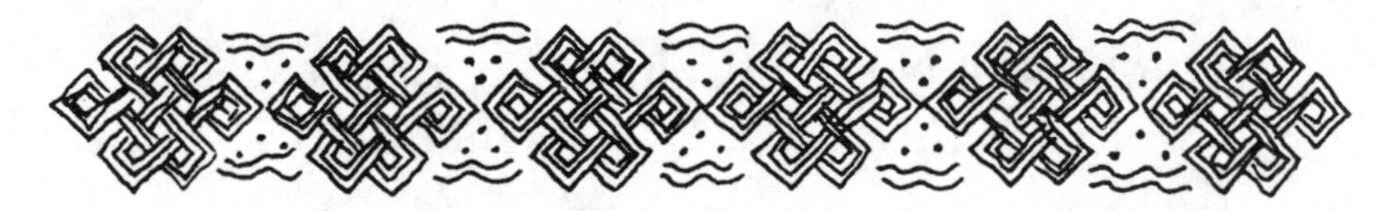

Steamed Li River Fish with Ginger and Spring Onion (Courtesy of Li Siu Chur, Executive Chef, Guilin Sheraton)

1	kg.	Li River fish
100	ml.	soy sauce
50	ml.	water
5	g.	coriander
5	g.	sugar
2	g.	seasoning
2	g.	salt
20	g.	fresh ginger
20	g.	spring onion
2	g.	chili powder
60	g.	Soy oil

Clean and gut the fish. Sprinkle the fish with salt and steam for approximately 7 minutes and place on a platter. Boil together water, soy sauce, sugar, seasoning, and salt. Pour the sauce around the steamed fish. Place fine shredded ginger, spring onion, and chili powder on top of the steamed fish. Heat up the oil until it is smoking and pour over the fish and serve.

4 servings

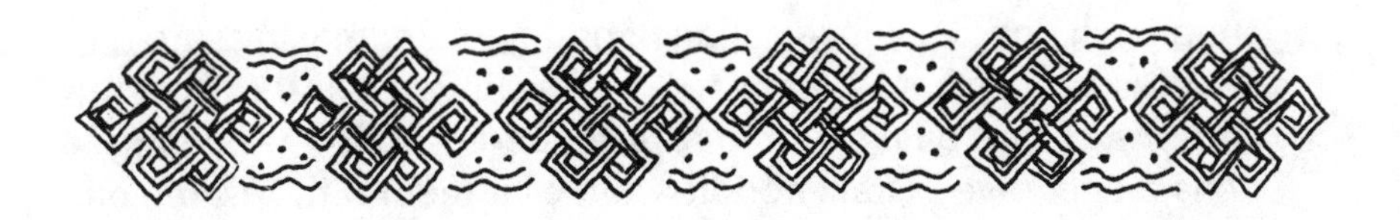

Shoulder Pole Carrying Noodles (Dan Dan Mein)

For Basic Noodles

3/4	lb.	egg noodles, fresh or dried
2	T.	sesame oil
2	t.	hot chili bean paste
1/4	C.	soy sauce
1	T.	vinegar
1	t.	roasted Sichuan peppercorns (*fagara*), crushed
1	C.	soup stock

For Meat Sauce

2	T.	cooking oil (safflower)
1/2	lb.	ground pork (beef may be substituted)
1	T.	ginger, minced
3		cloves of garlic, minced
2	T.	soy sauce
1	t.	sugar
1/4	C.	Shaoxing wine

Garnish (Optional, Use One or Both)

2	T.	chopped green onion
2	T.	chopped cilantro

Variations Have

dried shrimp (must be soaked overnight and trimmed)
shredded preserved vegetables

peanuts
sesame seeds
chili oil
additional garlic

Drop fresh noodles into a gallon of boiling water making sure the noodles are separated. Bring to a boil again, then add cold water and bring to a boil again. (For dried noodles follow the instructions on package.) Drain noodles and coat them with sesame oil. Set them aside in covered bowl to keep warm. Mix together the hot chili bean paste, 1/4 cup soy sauce, vinegar, crushed Sichuan peppercorns, and soup stock. Pour over noodles.

To Make the Meat Sauce

Heat cooking oil in a *wok* over a medium flame, stir in the ground pork so that it breaks up into fine morsels. Add ginger, garlic, soy sauce, sugar, and Shaoxing wine. Pour over noodle mixture and serve with green onion and cilantro. Add any of the variety ingredients to suit.

4 servings

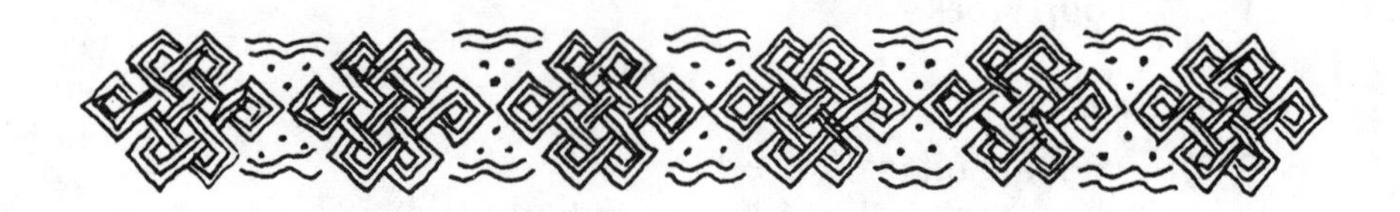

Cold Sesame Chicken (Bang Bang Ji)

1 3 lb. roaster
1 T. fresh ginger, minced
1 T. garlic, minced
1 t. roasted Sichuan peppercorns (*fagara*), crushed
1 T. sesame oil
1 T. hot pepper sesame oil
2 or 3 fresh bamboo shoots, sliced
3 T. soy sauce
2 T. Chinese sesame seed paste

1 T. Chinkiang vinegar
1 T. light brown sugar

Place whole chicken in a pot of water with ginger, garlic, *fagara* and bring to a boil. After it has boiled for about 10 minutes, remove the gray froth that forms with a skimmer. Cover and simmer the chicken for about 1 hour. Remove from heat and set aside. In a *wok*, heat the oils and add the sliced bamboo shoots. When they are tender, stir in the remaining ingredients. Add the chicken, either whole or cut up, and stir till all surfaces are well coated. Refrigerate up to 24 hours to chill before serving.

6 servings

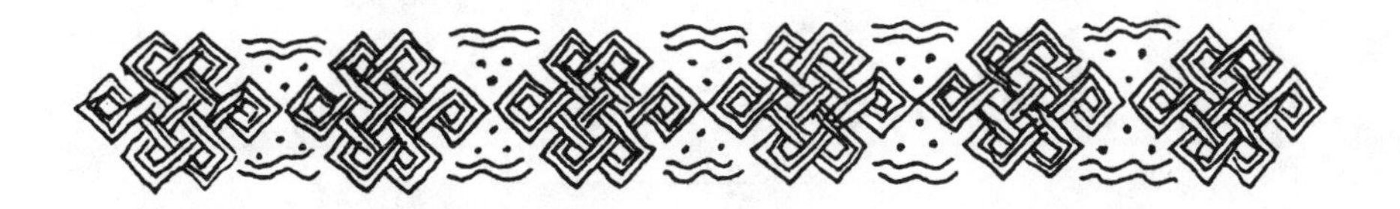

Twice-Cooked Pork (Wui Kuo Jou)

2 lb. uncured bacon (in one piece) (uncured pork shoulder or uncured ham may be substituted)
2 T. peanut oil (safflower oil may be substituted)
2 whole leeks
8 cloves garlic, minced
2-inch piece of fresh ginger, slivered
3 whole dried chili peppers
2 T. sweet bean paste
1 T. hot bean paste
2 t. sugar
1 T. soy sauce
1/4 C. Shaoxing wine

Simmer pork in just enough water to cover for one hour, then drain and cool. Slice the pork into pieces approximately 1/2-inch thick, then cut across into 2-inch pieces. Place the oil in a preheated *wok* and add the ginger, garlic, whole chili peppers, and leeks. Stir until the leeks are tender, add the pork, and continue stirring until the pork is well browned. Add the remaining ingredients, stir, and let simmer for about 5 minutes. *8 servings*

Variations

Add sweet red and/or green pepper with the pork in the *wok*. Or, stir in bite-sized pieces of spinach after pork has browned.

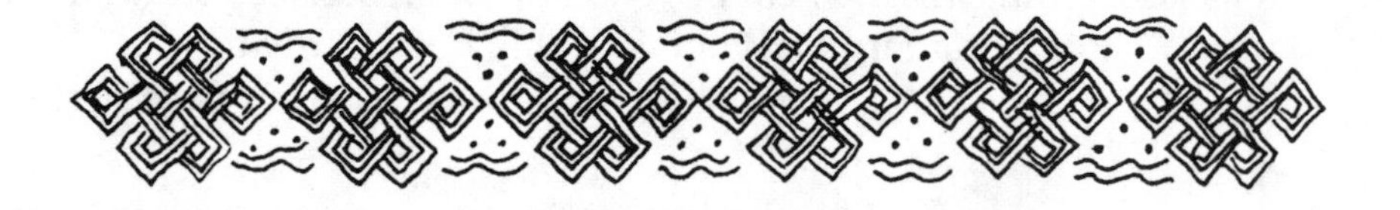

Sichuan Cucumber Relish (*Ma La Huang Kua*)

- 6 cucumbers
- 1 T. salt
- 4 cloves of garlic, minced
- 2 T. sesame oil
- 1 T. sugar
- 1 T. vinegar
- 1 T. hot pepper oil
- 1 t. crushed black Sichuan pepper

Cut the tips off of the cucumbers, slice in half lengthwise, and seed. Cut them into two-inch triangles and place them in a bowl with salt for 2 hours.

Drain and rinse. Mix together remaining ingredients and pour over cucumbers. If necessary add water to cover. Cover—will keep one week. *Yields 1 quart*

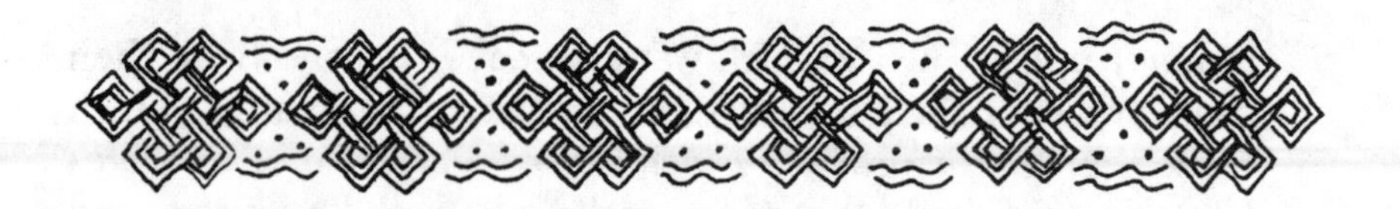

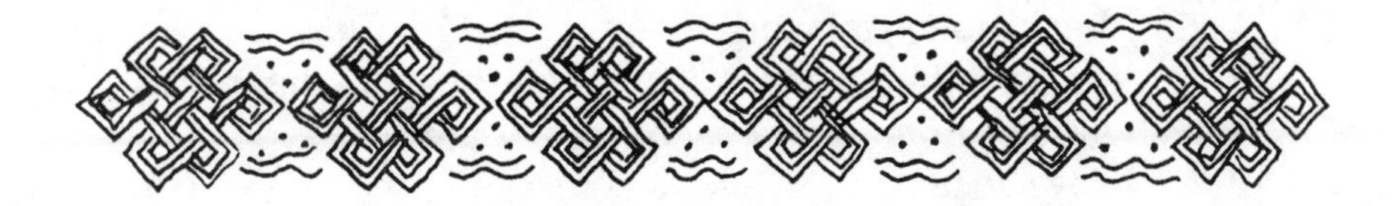

Eggplant Flavored Like Fish (Yu Xi' ang Qie Zi)

1	lb.	Chinese eggplant
4	T.	cooking oil (safflower)
1	T.	fresh ginger, minced
8		cloves garlic, minced
1	T.	hot bean paste
½–1	C.	soup stock
1	t.	sugar
2	T.	Chinkiang vinegar
1	T.	sesame oil
2	T.	scallions, chopped

Slice the eggplant into ¾-inch strips and fry in the cooking oil with the ginger and garlic. When the eggplant starts to brown and is slightly transparent, add the bean paste and stock mixed together. Cover and cook for 7 minutes. Remove the cover and add the remaining ingredients. Stir until well blended. Serve hot.

4 servings

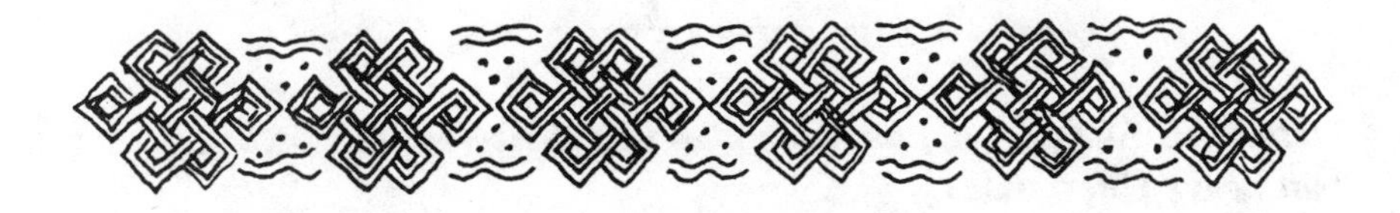

Dry-Cooked Yard-Long Beans (or String Beans) (Kan Pien Ssu Chi Tou)

2	lb.	yard-long green beans (or string beans)
1	C.	cooking oil (safflower)

1	T.	fresh ginger, minced
3	T.	dried shrimp, soaked for an hour (may be omitted)
1/4	lb.	ground pork (beef may be substituted)
2	T.	soy sauce
1	T.	Chinkiang vinegar
1/4	C.	hot water
1	t.	sugar
1	T.	scallions, minced

Clean, trim, and cut the beans into 4-inch pieces, or as desired. Rinse and drain the shrimp. Heat the oil in a *wok*. Fry the beans until they start to shrivel, or about 3 minutes. Remove the beans. Drain the oil from the *wok*, return 2 tablespoons of oil, and swirl with a *wok* spatula. Add the ginger, shrimp, and pork and stir until the pork is cooked. Add the beans and the remaining ingredients. Stir until quite dry. A dash or more of hot sesame oil may be added to taste. *8 servings*

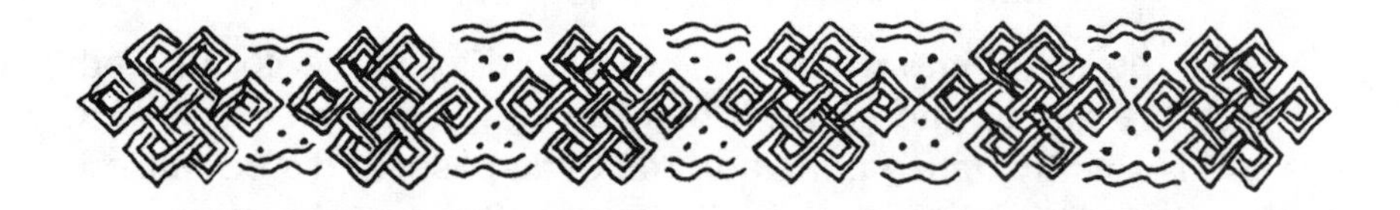

Sichuan Duck, Camphor and Tea Smoked (Chang Ch'a Ya)

Note: *This Should Only be Attempted in a Well-Ventilated Kitchen.* Do Not *Leave Unattended.*

1		Long Island duck—5–6 lb.
2	T.	salt
2	T.	Sichuan brown pepper

In small heavy skillet brown salt and pepper, then crush with mortar and pestle or spice mill. Rub the duck inside and out with the salt and pepper mixture and refrigerate, uncovered, on wire rack for 24 hours.

Three hours before serving preheat oven to 350°.
In large oven-proof *wok* place the following:

2 cups of wood chips, cedar, hickory or any aromatic cooking wood
½ C. tea leaves
1 C. raw rice
¼ C. orange peel

Make sure all ingredients are in the center of the *wok* and will not touch the sides of the oven. Place *wok* in oven until the wood chip mixture begins to smoke.

Then place the duck on a metal rack directly over the smoking mixture. Cover with a domed lid or a tent made of aluminum foil. Smoke the duck for 30 minutes. (Turn duck once after 15 minutes.) Remove the duck, cool and rub with a mixture of 1 tablespoon of minced ginger and 2 tablespoons of minced spring onion. Set up steamer and steam the duck for 2 hours. Remove the duck from steamer.

In clean *wok*, place 4 cups of cooking oil and, when hot, fry the whole duck 10 minutes, turn duck and fry 10 minutes more to make sure it is crisp on all sides. Serve immediately.

4 servings

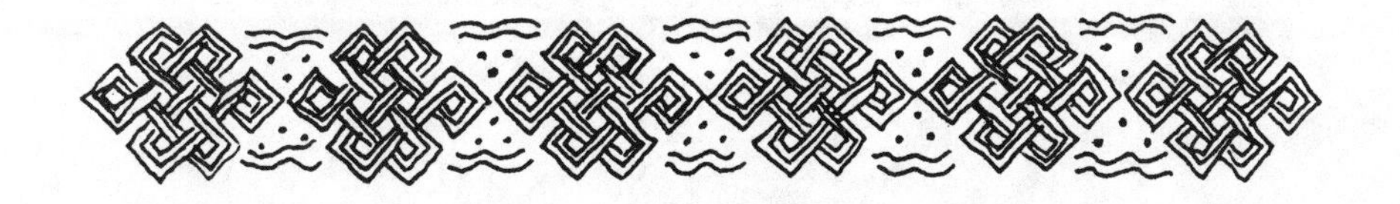

Spicy Chicken Breast and Peanuts (Tung An Ji)

2 whole chicken breasts, skinless and boneless
1 T. cornstarch
1 egg white
5 T. peanut oil
5 whole dried chili peppers
2 T. fresh ginger, minced

2	t.	roasted Sichuan peppercorns (*fagara*)
1/4	C.	raw peanuts, unsalted
1/4	C.	Chinkiang vinegar
1/4	C.	Shaoxing wine (dry sherry may be substituted)
2	T.	soy sauce
1	T.	sesame oil

Julienne the chicken. Mix the cornstarch and the egg white. Blend, then stir with the julienned chicken. Heat the oil in a *wok* and stir in chili peppers, ginger, peppercorns, and peanuts. When all are aromatic and lightly browned, add the chicken and stir until cooked. Add the remaining ingredients, except for the sesame oil. Stir until well blended. Serve on a warm plate with a few dashes of sesame oil. *4 servings*

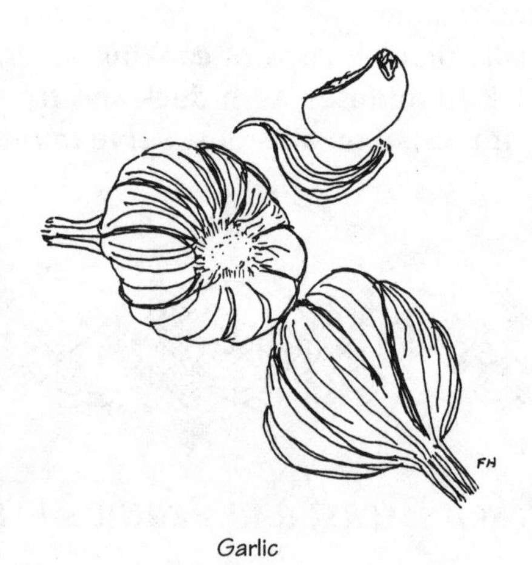

Garlic

6

Guangdong (Canton) and the South

Guangzhou, known better in English as Canton, is one of the largest and oldest cities in China and is located on the Pearl River, which flows through it. Though *pu tung hua* (Mandarin) is the official language throughout all of modern China, unspecified millions speak Cantonese in southern China and the rest of the world.

Guangzhou is sometimes called the "Goat City" because five ephemeral figures riding five goats entered Guangzhou in 1256 B.C.E. From the mouths of these five goats the five persons drew the first rice seeds. Guangdong province is still referred to as "the rice bowl of China." It is said, "Dress in Hangshou, marry in Sushou, die in Luzhou, but eat in Guangdong."

For a short period before the Han Dynasty, Guangzhou was the capital of the state of Nanue. It has been an international trading city since before the T'ang Dynasty. As early as 1000 C.E. Guangzhou was an international port, and ships from all of Asia and Europe traded there. By the nineteenth century, after the opium wars had closed other ports, Guangzhou remained open, and it was from there that large numbers emigrated to growing young countries like the United States.

Because of natural and man-made disasters, the area's food supply is on the mind of everyone who lives there. No food is taboo, and locals joke that the only thing with four legs they will not eat is a table. It has long been said that anything that flies, swims, or crawls is eaten, as long as it is fresh and prepared in a tasty way.

In Guangdong province Guangzhou and Chiu Chow (at the port of Shantou) have a rich and distinct culinary history that is famous the world over. In traditional households, two trips a day to the market continue to be the norm, ensuring that all food is at its freshest. Though chicken, pork, and other poultry are eaten, fish and vegetables are the sustaining ingredients of the cuisine, which is encouraged by Taoist and Buddhist tradition. It is from Guangzhou that many of the most familiar Chinese table sauces originate: chili sauce, mustard sauce, oyster sauce, and soy sauce.

The chefs of Chiu Chow believe that "You are what you eat." It is in Chiu Chow that the preparation and eating of bird's nests took on a mythic proportion, because the purified swallow saliva was thought to heal. This dish is on its way to extinction because of pollution and the precarious climb necessary to procure the nests from high cliffs. When the nests are combined with winter melon, ham, or chicken (or all three) they make for a savory soup; with sweetened almond paste, coconut, or other fruit they make an exceptional dessert. Another specialty, shark's fin soup, is the prize of a seafaring people with a strong sense of braving the ocean. A lesser-known specialty is pomfret smoked in Iron Buddha tea leaves, an elegant dish. Steamed dishes and quick *wok* cooking in peanut oil are prevalent, with the use of lots of vegetables and oyster and fish sauces. The regional specialties include the more familiar dishes of fried oysters, shrimp and crab balls, cuttlefish, clams, frogs, eels, carp, and whelk.

Chiu Chow sauces include the traditional ginger, but are also flavored with mixtures of fruit juices and spicy chilies that are mixed with oil and vinegar. Tangerines are used for sauces and also for jam, which is served with savory dishes. The tastes of special dishes tend to be very intense and therefore quite memorable. Oddities such as dog, monkey, snake, and pangolin are used more for medicinal benefits than as daily food. Southern Chinese cooking has strongly influenced the rest of China.

For three out of five people in the world, rice is the primary element in daily eating. In China the average consumption is close to 300 pounds per person per year in the areas where it is grown and almost that much throughout the rest of the country. The reason for this is that where rice is the dominant grain, few others are eaten; where it is not, rice is still included in the diet. One of its advantages over other grains is that it doesn't need processing. Of course it is often processed and eaten in different forms. By 2800 B.C.E. it was one of the "five sacred crops": barley, millet, rice, soybeans, and wheat. At that time there was also an eight treasure rice: eggs, ham, mushrooms, oil, onions, pork, rice, and soy sauce. There was also a "wild rice" (*cao son*) that is not a true rice, but closely resembles the grain cultivated by Native Americans.

The three basic types of rice used in China and elsewhere are: long-grain (*indica*) rice that tends to be light and fluffy when cooked or steamed; the short-grain (*japonica*) rice, stickier and starchier and used more frequently in Japan; and the short-grain glutinous or "sweet" rice which becomes very sticky when cooked and is opaque. Glutinous rice is used for *sushi*, stuffings, and desserts.

To prepare three cups of long-grain rice, rinse one cup of rice, drain, and place in a two-quart pot with two cups of water and bring to a boil. Boil for two to three minutes, cover the pan tightly, lower the heat, and simmer for fifteen minutes. Remove from the heat and let it stand, still covered, for ten minutes more. If you are using an electric rice cooker, follow the manufacturer's directions.

Often all three kinds of rice are combined to make rice porridge or *congee*. This is a favorite breakfast food, but is eaten at lunch, and dinner, or as an afternoon or late-night snack. This soupy dish varies in texture from a thick oatmeal-like consistency to a watery broth. It is made from raw rice in a proportion of ten or twelve times the water to rice, or from cooked rice in a ratio of five or six parts water to one of cooked rice. When made with raw rice, the cooking time is about two hours; and using cooked rice one hour.

Usually *congee* is cooked in water, but it can also be boiled with the bones of cooked chicken, duck, or pork. In Canton the *congee* tends to be cooked longer and becomes thinner than in other parts of China. It serves as a nutritious background for a wide range of savory tidbits that accompany it. The stress is on lightness accented with pickles, dried shrimp, *conpoy*, smoked fish, or squid. Garnishes such as scallions, peanuts, cilantro, ginger, pickles, and croutons made of fried dough sticks are toppings used in many places. These are usually added after the *congee* is cooked, but sometimes dried *dofu* skins are cooked along with it. This is also a good dish for leftovers. Spicy beef or lamb, cut into dice, or *dofu*, sprinkled with chopped cilantro, is a filling midnight snack. In China you can find *congee* at any price, and it is generally a delicious breakfast eaten streetside or in the armchair of a hotel dining room. "*Sik fan*" or "Eat rice" is the "*bon appetit*" of Guangzhou.

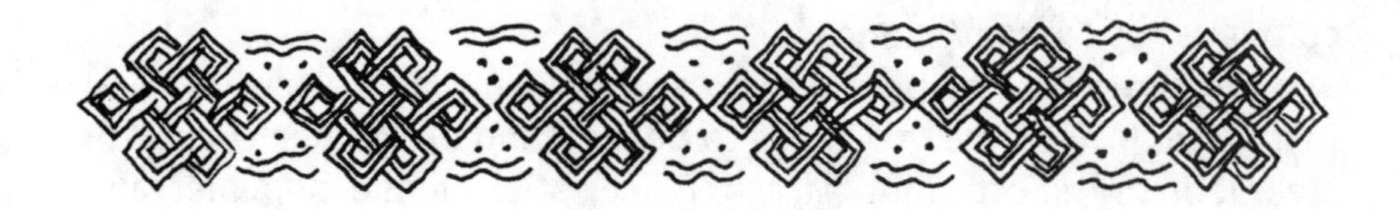

Congee (Yu Jook)

1	C.	short-grain rice
1	T.	peanut oil
10	C.	chicken stock
2	C.	water, if needed
2	t.	fresh ginger, minced

Rinse the rice in running water and drain. Mix the oil into the rice and set aside. Bring the broth to a gentle boil and stir in the rice and ginger. Stir and keep the liquid boiling for 10 minutes. Cover, lower heat, and simmer for 2 hours. Stir occasionally. If the mixture seems thicker than you like, gradually add up to 2 cups of water. Serve in warm bowls. Set out small plates with any or all of the following:

1/2	lb.	cooked chicken breast, cut in julienne
1/4	C.	chopped spring onions
1/4	C.	chopped fresh cilantro
1/2	C.	roasted peanuts
1/4	C.	Chinese pickles
1		fried dough stick (available in Chinese specialty stores)

The diner chooses the garnishes and places them on top of the *congee*.

4 servings

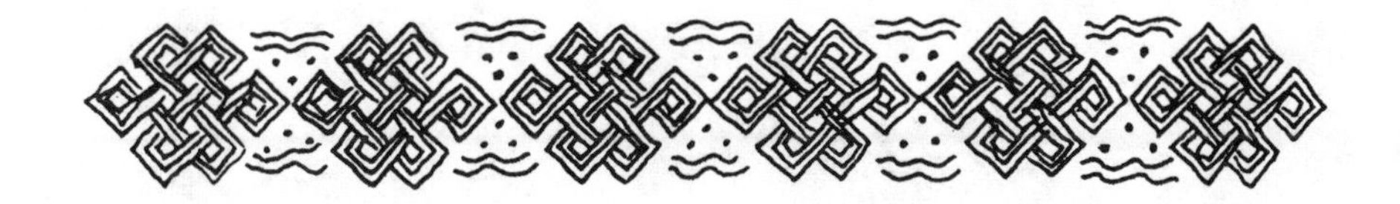

Cantonese Roast Pork (Char Sieu)

1½ lb. pork fillet

Marinade

- ¼ C. light soy sauce
- 1 t. fresh ginger, grated
- 2 cloves garlic, finely minced
- 2 T. Shaoxing rice wine (dry sherry may be substituted)
- 2 T. *hoisin* sauce

Basting Mixture

- ¼ C. Chinese maltose or honey
- ¼ C. hot water

Cut pork into strips approximately 6 inches by 1½ inches. Mix the marinade ingredients. Place the pork in the marinade, cover, and refrigerate for 3 hours or overnight. When ready to cook, heat the oven to 375°. Drain the pork and discard the marinade. Brush the pork with Chinese maltose or honey mixed with hot water. Using either special hooks designed for this purpose or a rack placed over a roasting pan, roast the pork for 20 minutes. Turn the heat up to 425°, baste, and roast another 10 minutes. The pork can be served hot or cold. Slice before serving. The cooked pork can be frozen and used in making dumplings, soups, and stir fries. Beef or turkey breast can be treated the same way.

6 servings

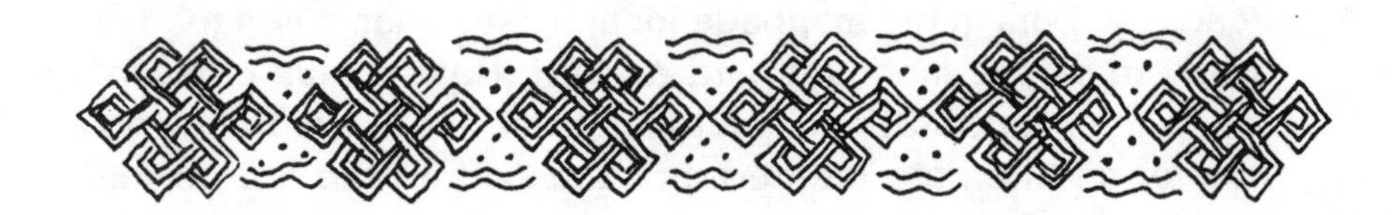

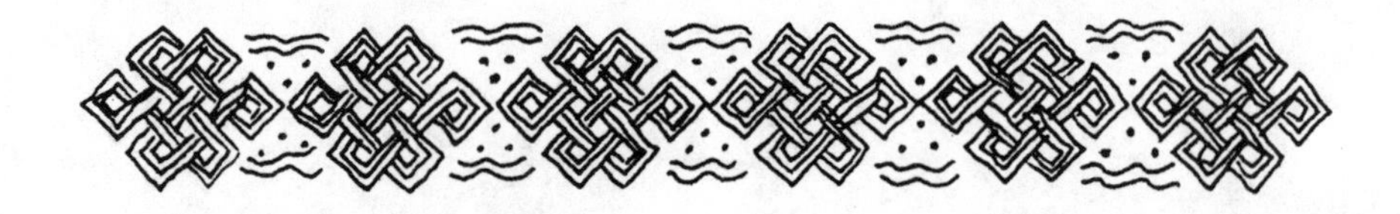

Sweet-and-Sour Pork (*Kulu Jou*)

Pork

1	lb.	pork tenderloin, cut in 1-inch cubes
3	C.	fresh pineapple, cubed
2		sweet green peppers, diced, with seeds and membranes removed

Marinade

2	T.	soy sauce
1	T.	Shaoxing wine (or dry sherry)
1/2	t.	salt
1		egg yolk
2	t.	cornstarch
1	T.	hot water

Sauce

1/4	C.	Chinkiang vinegar
1/4	C.	sugar
2	T.	Shaoxing wine (or dry sherry)
1	T.	soy sauce
1	T.	fresh ginger, minced
2	T.	tomato paste
3/4	C.	chicken or beef broth
6	C.	peanut oil for deep-frying pork in the traditional manner or 1/2 C. for stir frying

Place the pork in the marinade for at least 1 hour. When ready to cook, drain the marinade and discard. Heat 6 cups of oil in a deep fryer for traditional preparation or heat 1/2 cup of oil in a *wok* for an alternate method. Stir the pork in the hot oil until crisp. Remove the pork and discard the oil from the *wok*, leaving approximately 2 T. to stir fry the peppers and pineapple. Stir until cooked through. Add the sauce ingredients, stirring continuously. Add the pork and stir until well blended and hot throughout. Serve very hot. *4 servings*

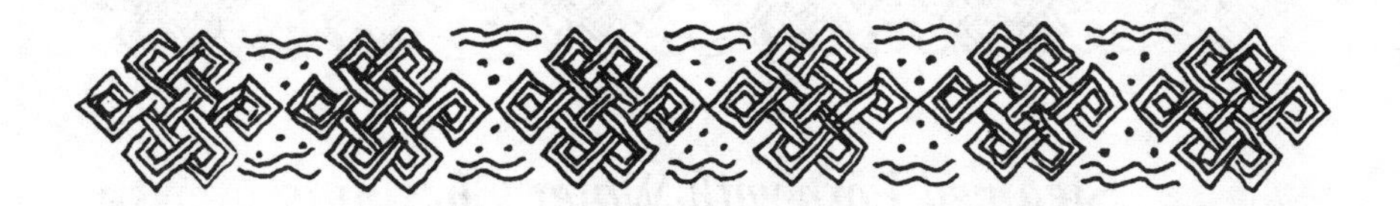

Easy Barbecued Spare Ribs

2 lb. spare ribs, in one piece if possible

Marinade

- 1/4 C. soy sauce
- 1/4 C. honey
- 1/4 C. Shaoxing wine or dry sherry
- 2 T. Chinese vinegar
- 1 T. *hoisin* sauce
- 1 t. fresh ginger, minced
- 1 t. fresh garlic, minced

Set the spare ribs in a shallow container. Mix the marinade ingredients until well amalgamated. Pour over the spare ribs and marinate for 6 hours or overnight. Turn the ribs occasionally to make sure they are well coated. When ready to cook, preheat the oven to 375°. Place a large roasting pan, half filled with water, on the bottom shelf of the oven. If possible, hang the spare ribs from the upper rack of the oven with S hooks. (They are sold for this purpose, but you may also find some at your hardware store.) Using the hooks, the ribs are over the pan, but not touching it. If this method does not suit you, the spare ribs may be roasted on a cake rack set directly on the upper oven rack.

Roast the ribs for 45 minutes. Turn the heat up to 425° and roast for another 15 minutes. Serve the ribs with assorted dipping sauces, such as plum sauce or hot sauce. *4 servings*

Steamed Pork with Water Chestnuts (Mar Tai Jing Ji Yook)

1	lb.	ground lean pork
1	C.	water chestnuts, fresh peeled (may use canned)
1/4	C.	spring onion, minced
1	T.	fish sauce
1/2	T.	light soy sauce
1	t.	sugar
2	t.	cornstarch
1	T.	cilantro leaves, chopped
		assorted Chinese pickles

Set a 10-inch or 12-inch steamer on a stove and bring water to a boil. Mix all the ingredients except the cilantro and pickles. Place the meat mixture in an 8-inch Pyrex pie pan and gently pat it out into an 8-inch circle. Set the pan in the steamer, cover, and cook for 30 minutes. Serve hot, topped with cilantro and pickles. *4 servings*

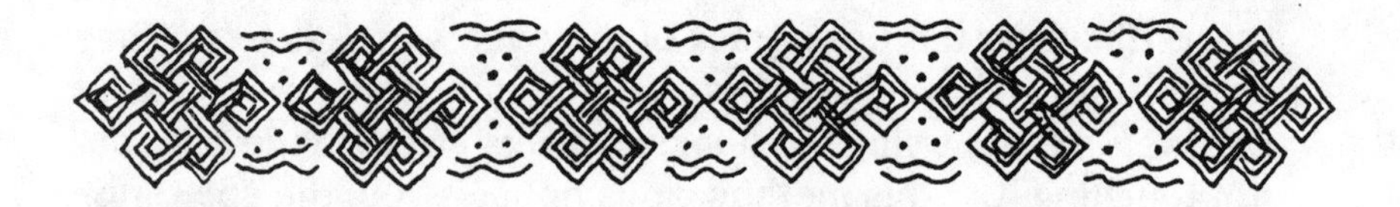

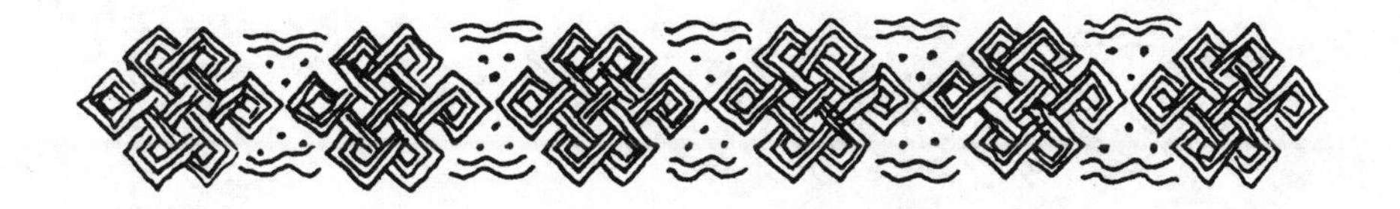

Beef with Oyster Sauce (Haoyu Niujou)

1	lb.	lean beef (London broil)
1	T.	soy sauce
1/4	C.	beef stock
1/2	t.	baking soda
1	t.	sugar
1	T.	cornstarch dissolved in 2 T. water
1	lb.	"yard-long" beans or string beans
2–4	T.	peanut or safflower oil
1	bunch	spring onions, cut in slivers
12		thin slices of fresh ginger
1	C.	water chestnuts, sliced
1/4	C.	Shaoxing rice wine (or dry sherry)
2	T.	oyster sauce
1	T.	water
1	T.	soy sauce
1	t.	sesame oil
1		pinch of salt
1		pinch of sugar

Slice the beef thinly and marinate in a mixture of soy sauce, beef stock, baking soda, sugar, and cornstarch for at least 1/2 hour. Cut the beans into 2-inch pieces and place them in boiling water for 2–3 minutes, then drain under cold water. Place 2 tablespoons of oil in a *wok* or skillet over high heat, and add the spring onions, ginger, and beef. Stir for 5 minutes. Add the beans and water chestnuts. Stir for another 5 minutes. Mix together the oyster sauce, soy sauce, water, sesame oil, salt, and sugar, and pour over the mixture. Stir until well blended. Serve immediately. *4 servings*

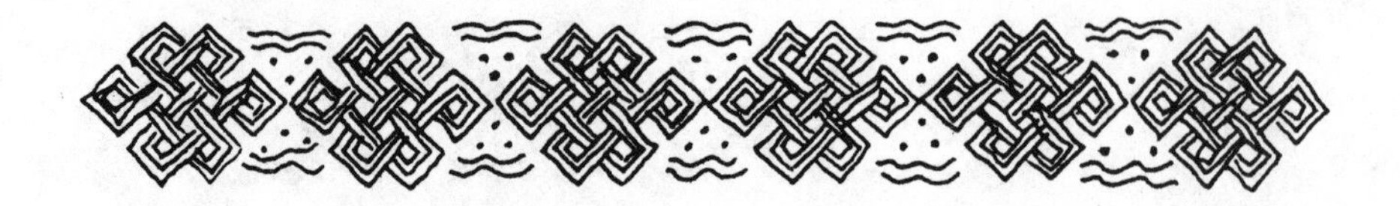

Abalone with Oyster Sauce (*Paoyu Cai Bao Pin*)

1	lb.	*bok choi*
3/4	C.	canned abalone (available at specialty stores)
4	T.	peanut or safflower oil
1	clove	garlic
1	t.	fresh ginger, minced
1–2	C.	fish or chicken stock
2	T.	Shaoxing rice wine (or dry sherry)
2	T.	oyster sauce
1	T.	light soy sauce
1		pinch of salt
1		pinch of sugar
1	T.	cornstarch dissolved in 2 T. water
1	t.	sesame oil
2	T.	cilantro leaves, chopped

Trim the tops and root ends of the *bok choi*, cut into 2-inch pieces, rinse, and dry. Slice the drained and rinsed abalone into 1/8-inch slices. Heat the peanut or safflower oil in a 10-inch or 12-inch *wok* or skillet. Add the garlic and ginger and stir. Add the *bok choi* and stir fry for 3 minutes. Add abalone slices. Stir fry for 30 seconds and add the remaining ingredients. Bring to a boil and continue stirring for 3 minutes. If additional liquid is needed, add up to 1 additional cup. Serve immediately with the chopped cilantro.

4 servings

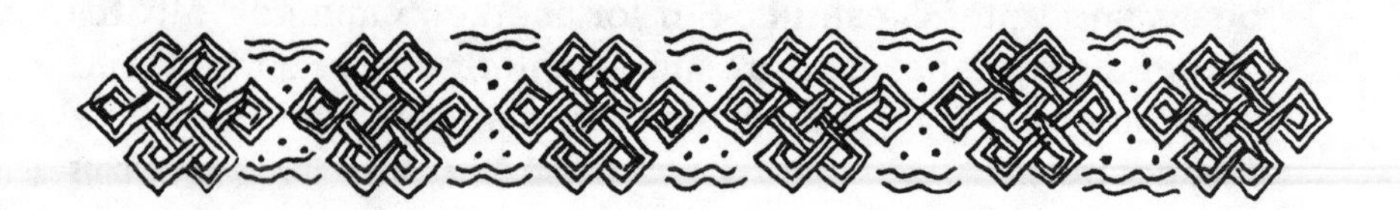

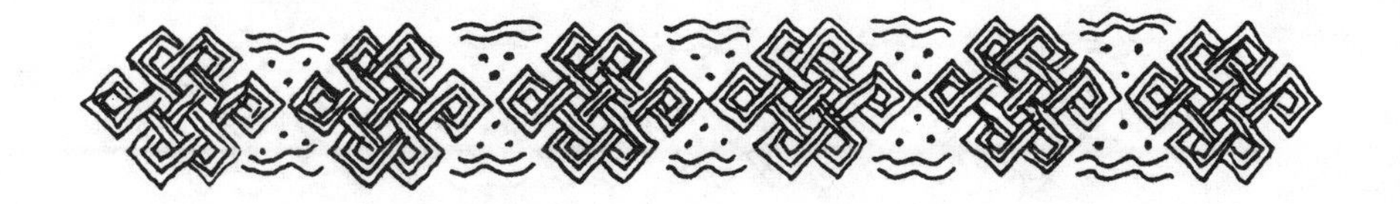

Shrimp in Black Bean Sauce

2	T.	peanut or safflower oil
1	lb.	shrimp, shelled and cleaned
1	t.	fresh ginger, minced
6		cloves of garlic, peeled and sliced
4		spring onions, cleaned and chopped
1	T.	fermented black beans, rinsed and slightly chopped
½	t.	sugar
1	T.	soy sauce
2	T.	Shaoxing rice wine (or dry sherry)
½		bunch of watercress, well rinsed, for garnish

Heat 2 tablespoons of the oil in a 10-inch or 12-inch *wok* or skillet, and stir in shrimp, until they are opaque (about 3 minutes). Remove and set aside. Add 2 more tablespoons of oil and stir fry the ginger, garlic, and spring onions for 2 minutes. Mix together the fermented black beans, sugar, soy sauce, and wine. Place the mixture in the *wok*, stir, and add shrimp. Stir until well blended and serve immediately. May be garnished with watercress.

4 servings

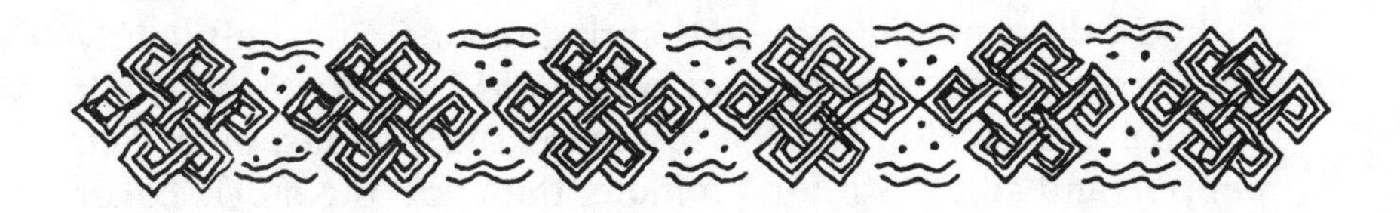

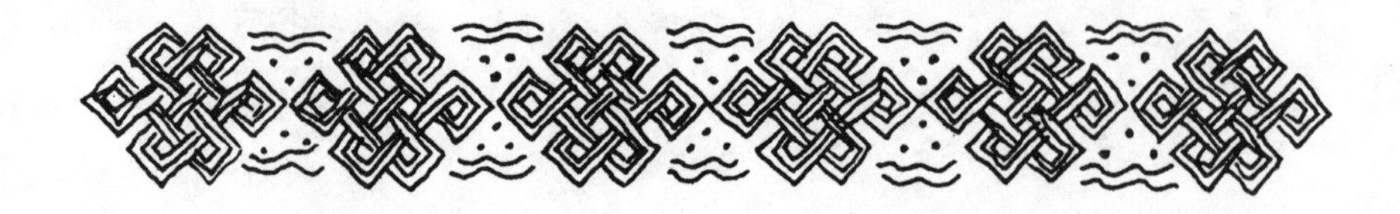

Lobster Cantonese (*Ch'ao Lung Hsia*)

1/4 C.	peanut or safflower oil
1 t.	fresh garlic, minced
1 t.	fresh ginger, minced
3	spring onions, chopped
1/4 lb.	ground pork
1 T.	fermented black beans, rinsed and chopped slightly
1 1 1/2–2 lb.	live lobster, cleaned, cut into pieces with the shell left on
1 T.	soy sauce
1 T.	Shaoxing rice wine (or dry sherry)
1	pinch of salt
2	pinches of white pepper
1/4 t.	sugar
1 C.	chicken stock (water may be substituted)
1 T.	cornstarch dissolved in 2 T. cold water
1	whole egg
1	egg white

Heat the oil in a 12-inch *wok* until hot. Lower the heat to medium and add the garlic, ginger, and spring onions. Stir until lightly browned and add the ground pork. Add the lobster and stir until it starts to color. Add the soy sauce, black beans, wine, salt, pepper, and sugar. Stir for 1 minute, then add the stock, cover the *wok*, and cook for 5 minutes. Uncover and add the cornstarch mixture. When the sauce is thick and clear, mix the egg and egg white together and pour over all in a thin stream, stirring to break up the eggs as they set. Serve immediately. 4 *servings*

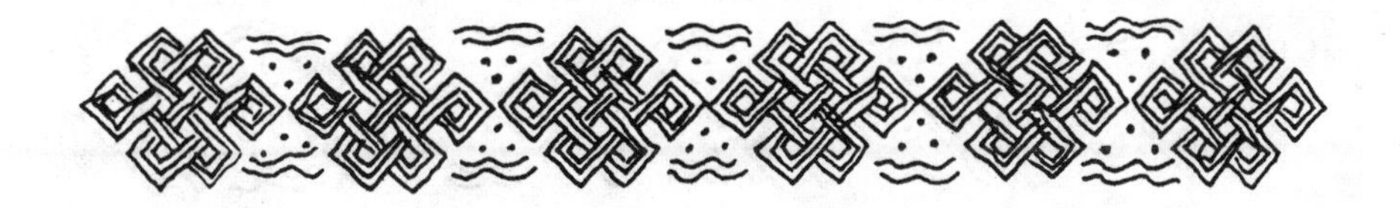

Chicken with Cashews (Cashew Gai Ding)

1	lb.	boneless chicken breast
1		egg white
1	T.	Shaoxing rice wine (or dry sherry)
1	T.	light soy sauce
1		pinch of salt
1		pinch of white pepper
½	t.	cornstarch
¼	C.	peanut or safflower oil
6	oz.	raw cashews
6		slices of fresh ginger, julienned
3		spring onions, cut in 2-inch pieces
½	lb.	fresh white mushrooms, quartered
¼	lb.	bamboo shoots
¼	C.	chicken stock or water
1	T.	oyster sauce
1	T.	Shaoxing rice wine (or dry sherry)
1		pinch of white pepper
1		pinch of sugar
½	t.	cornstarch, dissolved in 1 T. cold stock or water

Dice the chicken and place in a mixture of the lightly beaten egg white mixed with 1 tablespoon of the wine, soy sauce, salt, 1 pinch of pepper, and ½ teaspoon of the cornstarch. Let sit for 10 minutes. Heat the oil in a *wok* or skillet. Stir fry the cashews and remove. Add the ginger to the *wok*, stir, add the chicken, and stir for 2 minutes. Add the spring onions, mushrooms, and bamboo shoots. Stir fry until chicken is cooked, or about 5 minutes. Mix the stock, oyster sauce, wine, 1 pinch of pepper, sugar, and cornstarch mixture in a small bowl and pour over the chicken in the *wok*. Stir, add the cashews, and serve immediately. *4 servings*

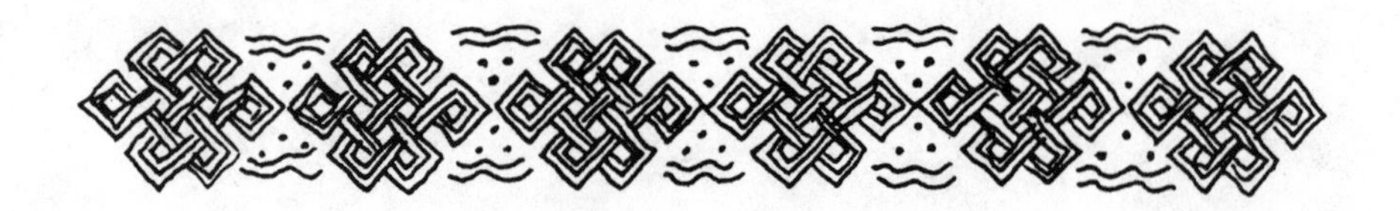

Chicken Liver *Stir* Fry

1	lb.	snow peas
1	lb.	chicken livers
1	T.	light soy sauce
1	T.	oyster sauce
1	T.	Shaoxing wine (or dry sherry)
½	t.	sugar
1	t.	cornstarch
¼	C.	peanut or safflower oil
1	t.	ginger, minced
1		bunch spring onions, cut in 2-inch lengths
		sprigs of cilantro for garnish

Rinse and string the snow peas. Blanch them in boiling water and drain under cold water. Clean the chicken livers, remove the membranes, and slice them. In a bowl large enough to hold the livers, mix the soy sauce, oyster sauce, wine, sugar, and cornstarch. Add the liver and stir. Heat the oil in a *wok* or skillet, stir fry the snow peas for 2 minutes, and remove. Stir fry the ginger and spring onions in the hot *wok* until the onions, are crisp. Add the livers and liquid and stir fry for 3 minutes. Add the snow peas and stir fry for another 2 minutes. Serve on a warm plate with the cilantro as a garnish. *4 servings*

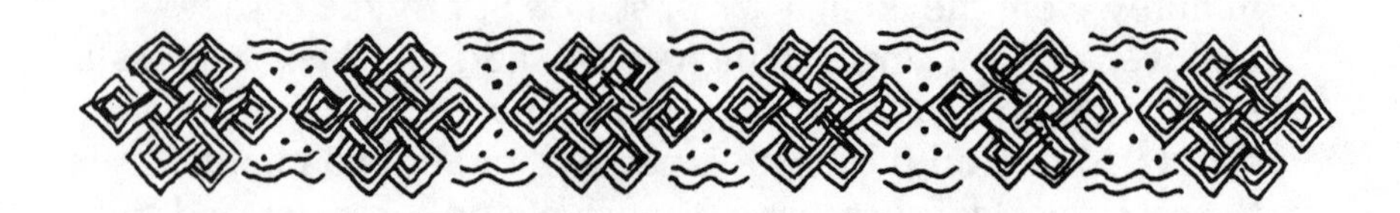

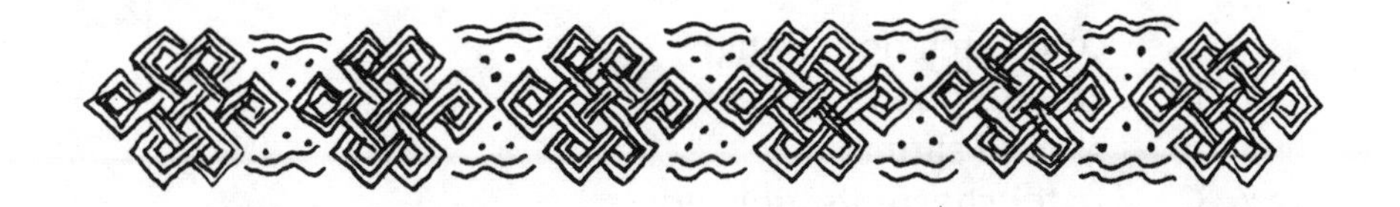

Minced Chicken and Corn Soup (Su *Mi* T'*ang*)

½	lb.	chicken breast
3		egg whites, lightly beaten
3		ears of fresh corn (frozen corn may be substituted)
7	C.	chicken broth or stock
1	T.	cornstarch dissolved in 2 T. cold chicken stock or water
		salt and pepper to taste
2	T.	Chinese ham, minced
2	T.	parsley, chopped

Mince the chicken breast and stir into the lightly beaten egg whites. Trim the kernels from the fresh corn, reserving any liquid. Bring the chicken broth or stock to a boil, add the corn and any corn liquid in bowl. Stir and bring to boil again. Add the chicken and stir until well distributed. Pour in a serving bowl and garnish with the minced ham and parsley. *4 servings*

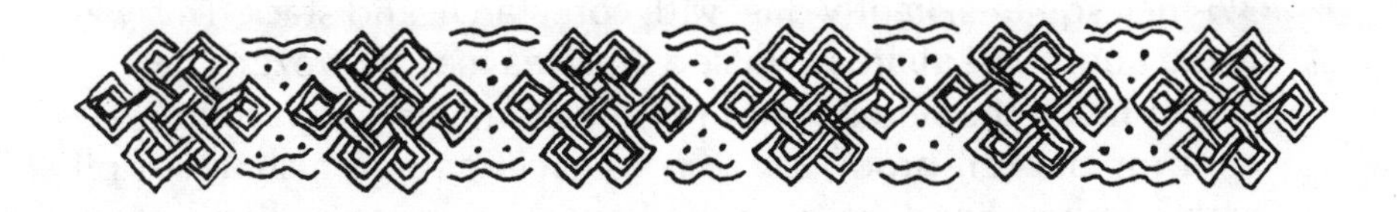

Wonton Soup (Hun *Tun* T'*ang*)

24		*wonton* wrappers: (frozen *wonton* may be substituted)
2	C.	flour
1		pinch salt
1		egg, lightly beaten
½	t.	peanut or safflower oil
½	C.	cold water

	cornstarch (for rolling)
1/2 lb.	ground pork
1/2 lb.	ground shrimp
1/2 C.	water chestnuts, minced
2	spring onions, minced
6	dried black mushroom caps, soaked, drained, and minced
1 t.	fresh ginger, minced
1/4 t.	white pepper
2 T.	light soy sauce
1 T.	sesame oil
8 C.	chicken broth
1 C.	*bok choi*, finely shredded
1 C.	Chinese spinach (*eng choi*), finely shredded
1/3 C.	spring onions, minced, for garnish

To make the *wonton* (frozen may be substituted), place the flour in a large bowl. Mix together the salt, egg, oil, and cold water. Pour into a well in the center of the flour and mix. Knead the dough for about 5 minutes, until very smooth. Let the dough rest for 10 minutes. Sprinkle the cornstarch on a pastry board and a rolling pin. Roll the dough until almost paper thin. If you have a small board, you may want to divide the dough in quarters. (A pasta machine may be used instead.) Cut the dough into 3 1/2-inch squares, lightly dust with cornstarch, and stack. This will make about 75 squares. Unused squares may be frozen.

To make the filling, combine the remaining ingredients except for chicken broth, *bok choi*, spinach, and garnish. Mix well with a fork or hands so that the flavors are evenly distributed. Place a generous teaspoon of the filling on each square. Fold the square corner to corner to make a triangle. Pinch the edges together, making sure that each is sealed. The outer ends of the triangle may be folded to meet as a small ring, if desired.

Bring a large pot of water to a boil and carefully drop in as many wonton as won't stick together. Bring the water to a boil again and remove the wonton with a slotted spoon. Set them on a slightly oiled platter. At this point they may be refrigerated or frozen.

If ready to use, bring the chicken broth, spinach, and *bok choi* to a boil and then gently add the *wonton*. Serve with a garnish of minced spring onions. *8 servings*

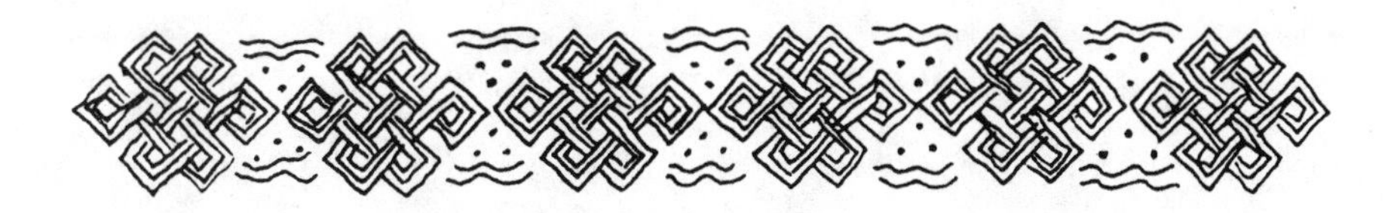

Cantonese Steamed Sponge Cake

6		eggs
1 1/4	C.	sugar
2	C.	flour
1	T.	baking powder
1/4	C.	peanut oil
1/4	C.	evaporated milk
1	T.	black sesame seeds

Beat the eggs and mix in the sugar until thick. Stir together the flour, baking powder, oil, and evaporated milk. Incorporate into the egg mixture. Line an 8-inch souffle dish (or similar 8-inch heatproof container) with plastic wrap lightly brushed with oil. Pour in the batter, and sprinkle with sesame seeds. Place the souffle dish in the steamer, cover it tightly, and steam over high heat for 40 minutes.

Remove the cake from the steamer. Cool briefly, cut into square or diamond-shaped pieces, and serve warm.

Variation: Stir 1/2 cup Chinese minced candied fruit (watermelon, lotus, jujubes, etc.) into batter before placing it into the souffle dish. *8 servings*

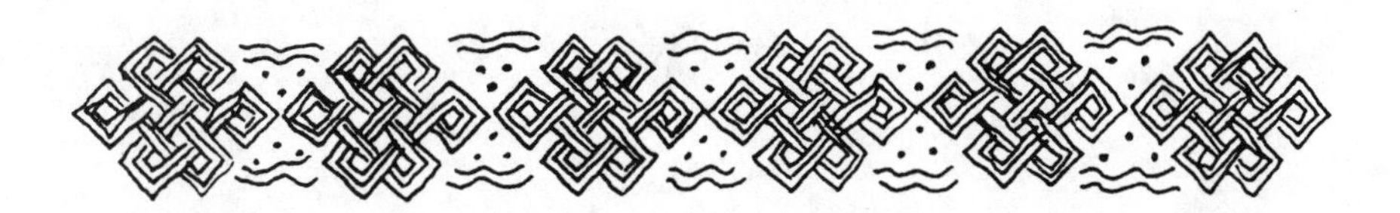

7

XIANGGANG (HONG KONG)

Almost Midnight

Flying low through the mountains into Hong Kong at night has to be one of *the* great landing experiences. Circling this twenty-first-century city skyline, flying past tall buildings with windows parallel to ours and so close we can look in, our enormous plane lands feet away from the water.

The green and watery patches surrounding Taipei Airport from the air were rice paddies and irrigation squares; the bright green rectangles interspersed with rectangles of water are tennis courts and swimming pools, still well lit at midnight. At this hour I am thrilled to be picked up at the airport, registered expeditiously at the Sheraton Hong Kong Hotel and Towers, and settled into a comfortable room. Looking out across the harbor from Kowloon, I sip hot tea and eat ripe fruit as I get my bearings.

Hong Kong, or as it is called in Mandarin, Xianggang, will be a semiautonomous "Special Administrative Region" on July 1, 1997 (the Year of the Ox). For the next fifty years, "One country, two systems" is to be the solution to maintaining the financial, commercial, and trade system as it stands. Not only is Hong Kong (in Cantonese, Heung Gong, or "Fragrant Harbor") Asia's most popular tourist destination, but it is constantly voted as one of the best places in the world in which to live.

Though clearly there will be change, it is hard to imagine Hong Kong much different than it is now. This world-class harbor has been filled through time with some combination of *sampans*, junks, tankers, freighters, sea planes, war ships, Western schooners, full-rigged clippers, small boats, hovercraft, cruise ships, ocean liners, ferries and pleasure craft. In 1849 the junk Keying traveled to New York, then London, popularizing things Chinese as it went. The ship was dismantled in Liverpool and the teak it was made of was used for ferry boats; bits of bamboo and tea crates were turned into *chinoiserie*, starting a craze that has yet to subside.

Nothing seems to happen in Hong Kong that is not accompanied by food. British, American, French, and Dutch settlements are well ensconced. Since early in the nineteenth century, merchant companies from Portugal, Germany, Italy, and India have had offices here. They brought cooks and drink: claret, champagne, port, and sherry. Dinners of shark's fin soup, roast beef, and Yorkshire pudding are no more unusual here than the laws of *feng shui* being observed by multimillion dollar constructions.

Feng shui is the geomancy of wind and water that rules how both public and private buildings should be positioned, to ensure the most auspicious relationship to their natural environment. Built according to this principle of harmony is the Bank of China, the largest skyscraper outside of the United States; it is the centerpiece of the city's financial landscape and also acts as a backdrop for full-moon picnics and cemetery banquets. Hong Kong has a history of always being ready for the new by changing, adding, incorporating, and letting go. The city is close to being in perpetual motion.

Hong Kong's history begins with the Yueh, a Stone Age tribe. They were originally fishermen who then expanded inland to establish farming. Their society grew stable enough to trade with the Han Dynasty (206 B.C.E.–221 C.E.). By the Sung Dynasty (960–1279 B.C.E.), Hong Kong was well settled. Trying to escape from Kublai Khan, the "wandering Sung court" set up a temporary palace in Kowloon. In Cantonese the name is Kow Lung or "Nine Dragons." In 1279 troops attacked the Sung in Hong Kong and the short-lived Yuan Dynasty (1280–1368 A.D.) under the Mongols came into being. They are remembered with respect in Hong Kong because they prohibited pearl fishing because so many divers had died.

When the Ming Dynasty (1368–1644 C.E.) overcame the Yuan, they held Hong Kong and its surrounding territory in contempt and neglect, resulting in a status quo of lawlessness and pirating. Next, the

Manchu invaded and the Qing Dynasty was established (1644–1911 C.E.). It brought about cruel disjunctions in civil life. People were pushed back from the coast and forbidden to return under pain of death. In 1841 Hong Kong was occupied by the British. In the Treaty of Nanking China ceded the thirty-two-square-mile island to Britain. Its feudal villages rank with malaria, typhus, dysentery, and cholera and its dealings in opium and slaves seem as remote a part of history as our civil war and its epidemics.

Blockades, boycotts, strikes, and riots established strong-knit factions throughout the country. In the late 1930s many people from southern China fled to Hong Kong to escape the Japanese invasion, only to be sent back when the Japanese took Hong Kong in 1941. In 1948 when the war was over, many people returned to Hong Kong and were soon followed by millions more who fled south for political reasons.

Through the vicissitudes of Chinese policies and the Korean and Vietnam wars, Hong Kong emerged by 1970 as an independent and strong financial and trade market. Because it is one of the best harbors in the world, ship-building and maintenance are big industries here and ships of every description ply the water. Publishing, printing, building, and manufacturing were given a remarkably free reign, in part due to the work of the "Independent commission against corruption." Honoring the tradition of *feng shui*, the infrastructure was expanded and cared for, with great respect for the natural terrain and its resources.

The Star Ferry Company has sent ferries across the harbor between Tsim Sha Tsui on the southern tip of Kowloon and central, old Victoria on Hong Kong island since 1868. The green-and-white diesels make the ten-minute crossing, twelve knots, 400 times each day. Some of the snacks and beverages sold at the ferry terminals are the same sort that have been there since its beginning, but now, of course, espressos, capuccinos, lattes, and biscotti are available.

Friday

I start the day having coffee with Heinz Schmeig, executive chef of the Hong Kong Sheraton. His background and experience are international: an early apprenticeship in Germany and then London, followed by long stints in Dubai and Cairo, where he became an executive chef. Now at the Sheraton in Hong Kong for seven years, he holds one of the most exciting jobs in the food industry—he is in charge of all the Hong Kong Sheraton's restaurants. He is familiar not only with traditional Asian cuisines, but also others that interact with them. As Western food is influenced by Chinese ingredients and style, they, too, are influenced by the West. Some exchanges of ingredients make for an exciting enrichment. Of course in hotels, as with all established restaurants, there is the dilemma of guests coming back after a few years and wanting to sample a memorable dish. There must always be a balance between the set menu with its signature dishes and daily specials that vary. At the Celestial Court Restaurant, guest chefs from specific regions also come to ply their local cuisine. There are fixed menus that are regional: Sichuan, Hunan, etc. The *à la carte* menu is Cantonese. The chef and the restaurant manager plan the menu and have total control; the executive chef does tastings for pleasure and quality control. Mr. Schmeig is pleased to see such an active and crowded culinary atmosphere. "When many people do things well and are creative you get some delicious new dishes added to the traditional field," he says. "There are, of course, a lot of terrible experiments when people jump on the bandwagon, but overall it is good for the profession to take some chances."

I tour the kitchens and pantries. Everything is tile and stainless steel. Computers track everything. Just as I am thinking it is all too twenty-first century, I am led through the cold storage room and given a down coat and gloves to put on. We enter a freezer room where a sculptor in a down coat and gloves is creating a traditional figure in ice, a sculpture that is larger than life and twice as intricate. It is the story of the dragon pearl. A dragon holding a pearl in his mouth is sitting on a chariot drawn by a flying horse. The sculptor has been at it a week and it will take another to finish.

Next I meet Stephen Wong at Hong Kong Tourism's new office in the Citicorp Center. He is not only a director of tourism, but a restaurant critic who writes about restaurants worldwide. We go to the Snow Garden Restaurant on the ground floor of 233 Electric Road in North Point. I look at the menu while he orders.

He is smiling and in deep conversation with the waiter, so I know beforehand I am in for a treat. The tea he orders is jasmine and I fear it will be too perfumed, but it is delicately scented and refreshes rather than dominates the palate. The first dish is dried bean curd sheets cooked like goose: layered, shredded, and fried like *filo*. They are crisp outside and flavored in the soft center. The second is tendon with sinew in brown sauce. The fish dishes are yellow croaker and cloud fungus in fermented rice wine mixed with vinegar and sugar, and then a dish of fish maws and *jin hua* ham. Though the fish maws are cooked simply in a white sauce with mushrooms and *bok choi*, each morsel is tasty and the air-dried ham literally melts in your mouth. We have crab soup and steamed dumplings, each served on a carrot slice with a tiny bud cut from a carrot to top it. The second soup is a rich, clear broth with sturdy bean curd cut into vermicelli and slivers of vegetables and mushroom. It is simple and satisfying. Dessert looks like sweet beans, but they turn out to be tiny fool-the-eye shaped dumplings made from glutinous rice. They are served in a fermented rice broth flavored with cassia and orange sections. I try to show restraint, but this is comfort food at its best.

Born in Hong Kong, he is very knowledgeable about both regional food and world cuisine, as he first worked for various airlines and has been with Hong Kong Tourism for many years. We talk about how food is part of everyday life in ways that are ignored by most people, and how people go to extremes, becoming either fearful or greedy, and miss the point of integrating the food for its humanness. He is a good eating companion.

I ask him a bit about the Hakka, the "guest families" as the nomads of an older China were called, who traveled from north to south and camped as the guests of other tribal families. The Hakka carried with them pickles, making salt-baked chicken, bone marrow with mushrooms, beef balls, fish balls, and other hearty, tasty fare.

Neolithic families were fishing off sandbars in what is now the archipelago of Hong Kong. Today most full meals here have at least one fish dish, and every chef worth their keep can cook fish to a millisecond. It is estimated that 150 tons of fish are consumed in the 400-square-mile territories daily. Though Tin Hau is still the Taoist goddess of fishermen, her main intervention is to bring safety in storms.

Modern technology, along with first-hand knowledge handed down for generations, plays the decisive role in the catch. Many of the beautiful old junks have been equipped with the most modern electronic equipment available and are worth millions. As descendants of "sea gypsies," the Tanka and Hoklo often referred to have settled down and number among the most successful Hong Kong fishermen. In addition to the area's natural resources, not much about the fish supply is left to chance. Aquaculture is everywhere, and on Lamma Island it is the main industry. Favorite fish include carp, garoupa, pomfret, sole bream, and mullet. It is, of course, the carp, with its attributes of perseverance and ambition, that has great cultural significance. After all, the urge to prosper is important to all immigrants, and free enterprise is common to settlers all over the globe. Hong Kong's population has grown through immigration, and it is only in the last ten years that well over half the census of six million were born in Hong Kong.

Mr. Wong puts me in a cab for the tram at the base of Victoria Peak. There has been a tramway up to Victoria Peak since 1888, when the train's engine was steam powered. Now, as then, the walk around Victoria Peak feeds the senses. This is not regarded a world-class destination for no reason. The fluttering butterflies are the kind animators draw to make people smile.

In the Pearl River tidal basin, Hong Kong, surrounded by bright blue-green water, is the largest island of the more than 200 that make up this archipelago. Superlative adjectives generally belie the truth, but the exhilaration here inflates one's vocabulary. Along the walkway at the peak, street vendors and food stalls are busy as are the stores and restaurants. The Häagen Daz store has the same selections offered everywhere. Five of the top ten McDonald's restaurants in the world are in Hong Kong.

I have dinner at the Celestial Court at the Sheraton. We have Iron Buddha tea which, it is said, grows so high up in the mountains that only monkeys can scramble up to pick it and take it down to their keepers. It is pale and subtle.

We have the best shark's fin soup I have had: light, not gelatinous, and with the addition of red vinegar, it is perfection. It is important that the soup not be served in shallow Western soup bowls in which it quickly chills and loses its rich texture and aroma. The deep, covered soup bowls of varying sizes used here are something that some Western restaurants would benefit from using. We also have shrimp and bean pods in a taro nest that is very fresh and pretty, then pigeon and *dofu* in brown sauce. We get rice and some special sauces; one is a mixture of dried shrimp, dried scallops, garlic, and chili paste that is quite good. Some of the side dishes are bland, such as the warm bean sprouts.

At 9:30 I meet an acquaintance to go to the Tsim Sha Tsui *daipaidong* (food stalls) and night market off the Haiphong Road. For centuries *daipaidong* have fed the itinerants of Hong Kong: immigrants, seamen, wanderers, merchants, tradespeople, artists, religious and political emissaries, missionaries, and pirates. It is a busy web of streets, alleys, store fronts, and stalls with merchandise. Here one can see cakes, dumplings, herbs, fruit, kitchenware, gaudy plastics, antiques, red and gold calligraphy, and and neon signs against the beautiful opaque night. Cures and good fortune are being offered, along with herbal teas and medicines, both packaged and brewed. Here are fortune tellers using birds, *chien shih* divining sticks, and palm readings and astrologers using charts and talismans. Musicians whose ages seem to range from ten to one hundred sing classics and folk music. Groups sing pop tunes accompanied by as many as five musicians. There are opera singers with small stages and one with an electric pippa (an ancient stringed instrument).

Locals and tourists eat together at the outside tables of the seafood stalls that sell live clams, crabs, shrimp, and abalone of every description. These items are cooked, sauced, and served to your order. A small taste proves them delicious. Many fish and shellfish are dried, salted, pickled, or preserved in some fashion. Oysters, abalone, jellyfish, and shark's fins are among them. Small whole fins in your soup mean you are being treated very well indeed.

I am surprised that, instead of the cloth and paper banners usual in outdoor markets, this one has a vast assortment of neon signs, decorative lights, and illuminated logos. An enormous indoor market with food stalls made from corrugated tin and canvas is crowded with people seated at at least one hundred tables. Portable kitchens line the walls and in them cooks tend to steaming pots.

We turn a corner and the street is lined with "proper restaurants," each with about ten to fifteen tables. There are noodle places, *congee* places, and more. Specialists abound. Though dog meat is forbidden in Hong Kong, snake and other traditional exotica are not, because they have such a long history. People are everywhere as we walk toward the water to a monsoon shelter. It is almost midnight and even the side streets are full of people.

The Next Morning

I go out and find a street breakfast of crullers (*yao tiao*) and *char siu*, a sheet of noodle wrapped around honey-glazed pork.

It is hard to find individual food *sampans* near the city, but they can be found in Aberdeen. Though shuttle launches leave from the main pier, I have walked far from there, and as I stand looking out towards the water, a lone mariner offers me a lift in his *sampan* to go to the large floating restaurants that have replaced the food *sampans*. The Jumbo and the Sea Palace are the largest of these with several decks that contain works of art, chandeliers, large fish tanks, and a cast of thousands to man the tanks, the tables, the kitchen, and the gift shops.

The restaurants on stilts in Lei Yue Mun at the eastern end of Victoria harbor offer unusual services. Select your seafood from any of the local fishmongers, and they will prepare it to your order while you relax and look out over the water.

Hong Kong has been and certainly continues to be Chinese, through thick and thin. That being said, it is necessary to remark that there is also an international culinary palate that is impressive. Some of the Japanese and Indian restaurants cannot be topped. The Thai food is excellent. People here also talk about the "new cooking," which tends to be Pan-Asian. But there are many East-West combinations as well. By and large, though, the cuisine emphasizes the distinct flavors of the regions of China with a predominance of Cantonese cooking, satisfying the palates of everyone for whom gourmanderie is an avocation.

The first three recipes that follow are courtesy of Heinz Schmieg, executive chef of the Sheraton Hong Kong Hotel and Towers.

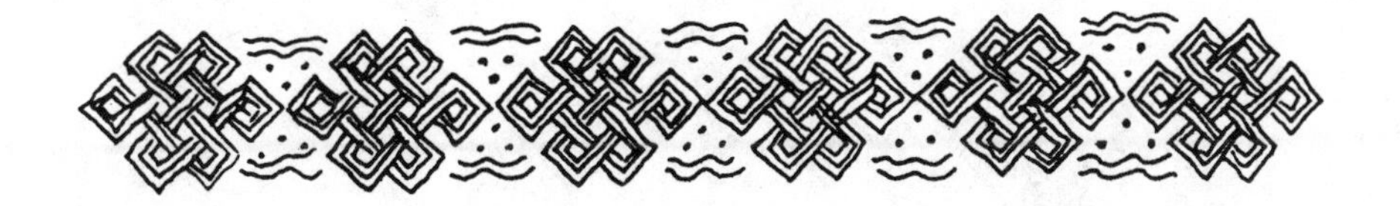

Pork Chops and Lemon Sauce

1	lb.	pork cutlets
1		large carrot
1		large stalk of celery
1		lemon
		juice of 1 lemon
3	T.	sugar
3	T.	chicken bouillon powder
2		egg whites
2	T.	cornstarch
4	T.	cooking oil
2	T.	parsley, minced

Rinse the cutlets and pat dry. Slice the carrot, celery, and lemon. Place them in a saucepan with 2 cups of water. Simmer for 30 minutes and strain, reserving the liquid. Return the liquid to the pan and add the lemon juice, sugar, and bouillon powder. Mix well and set aside. Dip the cutlets in the egg white and cornstarch mixed together. Heat the oil in a *wok* or skillet and fry the cutlets. Serve on a warm platter with the sauce and garnish with parsley.

4 servings

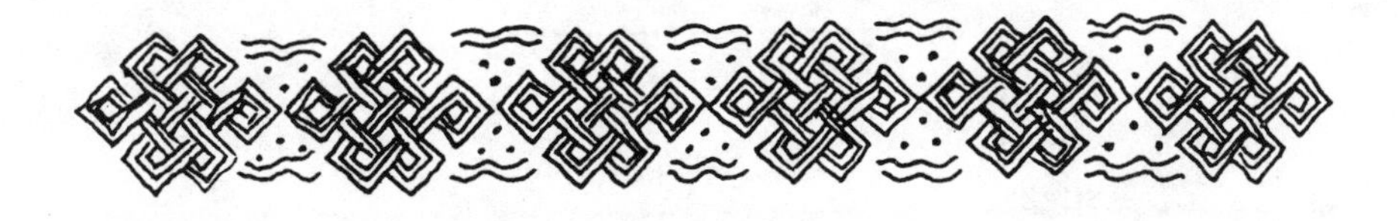

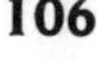

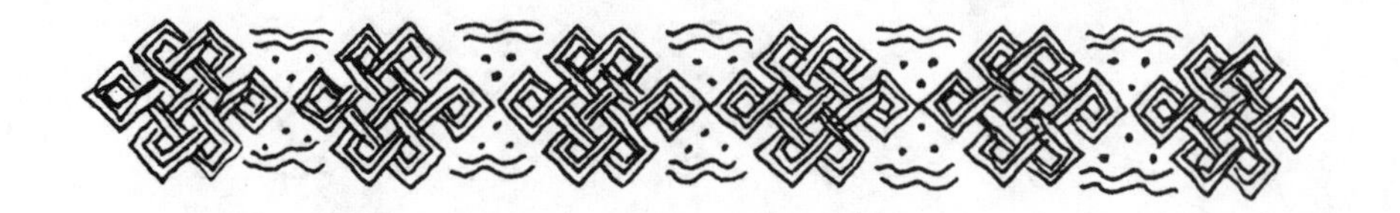

Sichuan Shrimp

1 lb. large shrimp
2 T. peanut oil
2 cloves of garlic, minced
2 T. shallots, minced
1 T. bean paste
1 t. sugar
1 T. cilantro (fresh coriander), chopped

Blanch the shrimp in boiling water for 1 minute, then drain and reserve. Heat the peanut oil in a *wok*, add the garlic and shallots, and stir till aromatic. Stir in the bean paste and sugar. Add the shrimp and saute for about 3 minutes. Arrange on a platter and serve garnished with chopped cilantro. *4 servings*

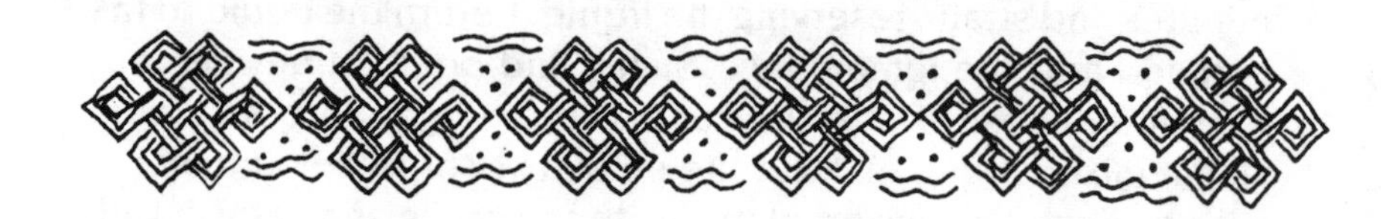

Shrimp and Squid Combination

1 lb. shrimp
3/4 lb. squid
1 T. sugar
2 t. sesame oil
1 egg white, lightly beaten
1 T. cornstarch
2 t. ginger juice

2	t.	Shaoxing wine
1	t.	light soy sauce
3	T.	cooking oil
5		slices of fresh ginger
2		cloves of garlic, minced
1/2	C.	shallots, chopped
1	t.	salt
1		carrot, sliced and blanched
3/4	C.	celery, sliced

Sauce

1	t.	salt
1	T.	cornstarch
1	t.	Shaoxing rice wine
2	T.	sugar
1	T.	soy sauce
1	t.	sesame oil
2	T.	chopped parsley, as garnish
1		carrot, sliced thinly, as garnish

Peel and devein the shrimp and wash in cold water. Dry the shrimp and marinate in 1/2 teaspoon sugar, 2 teaspoons sesame oil, 1 lightly beaten egg white, and 1 tablespoon cornstarch. Wash the squid tubes, cut each lengthwise, and open into a square. Score the squid in a cross-hatch. Marinate it in 2 teaspoons ginger juice, 1 teaspoon Shaoxing wine, 1 teaspoon light soy sauce, and 1/2 teaspoon sugar.

Place the cooking oil in a *wok* and stir fry the ginger, garlic, salt, and shallots. Add the shrimp and squid and stir fry at high heat. Add 1 teaspoon of wine, celery, and carrot and stir fry. When done, add the sauce ingredients. Arrange on a platter and garnish with chopped parsley and carrot slices. *4 servings*

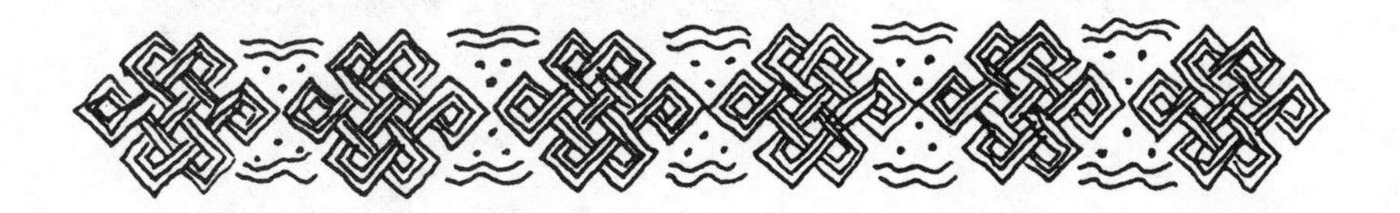

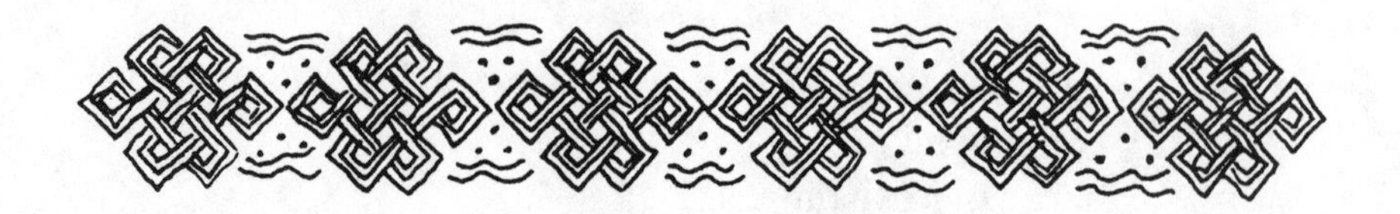

Hot-and-Sour Soup

6		dried black mushrooms, soaked, rinsed, and sliced fine
2		blocks of *dofu*, sliced thin
1/2	C.	bamboo shoots, cooked and sliced thin
1/2	lb.	cooked pork butt, cut into matchsticks
1	qt.	fresh or prepared chicken stock
1/2	t.	salt
1/4	t.	white pepper
1	T.	soy sauce
2	T.	white vinegar
2	T.	cornstarch mixed with 4 T. cold water
1		egg, lightly beaten
3		spring onions, cut into matchsticks, as garnish
2	t.	sesame oil
1/2	t.	hot chili oil (or to taste)

Set out the sliced ingredients. Bring soup stock, mushrooms, salt, pepper, and soy sauce to a boil. Add the bamboo shoots and pork. Simmer for 5 minutes. Add the *dofu* and vinegar. Stir and add the cornstarch mixture. Stir till the soup starts to thicken and add the lightly beaten egg. Serve garnished with spring onions and sprinkled with the oils. *4 servings*

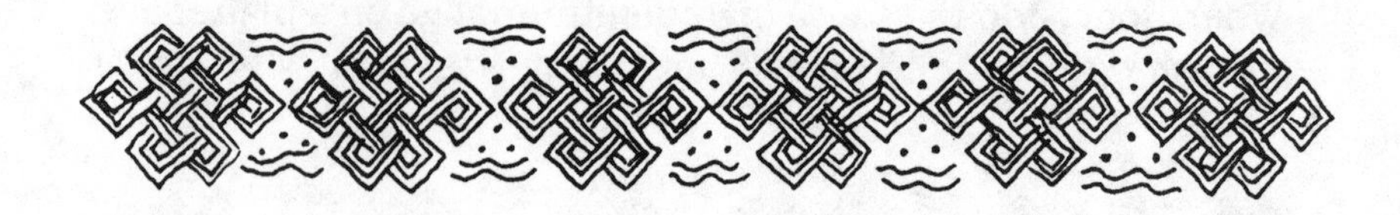

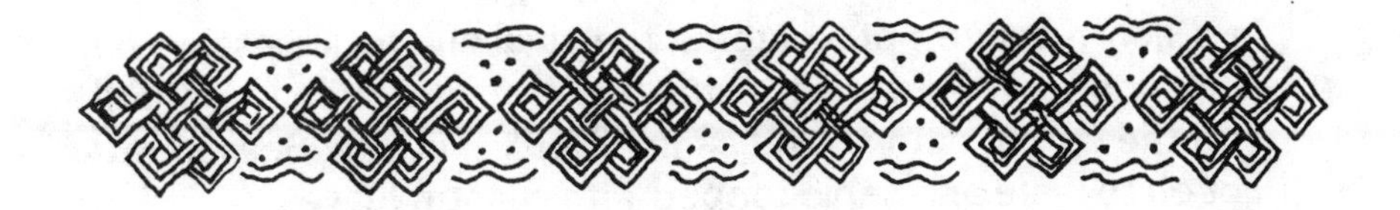

Winter Melon Soup

10 C. water
1 small chicken, cut in eighths
10 slices of fresh ginger, minced
5 dried Chinese black mushrooms, soaked, rinsed, and cut in wedges
1½ lb. winter melon, cut in 2-inch chunks
2 oz. dried shrimp, soaked for 1 hour

Combine the water, ginger, chicken, and mushrooms. Bring to a boil and simmer for 1 hour. Remove the chicken and debone. Cut the chicken into 2-inch pieces and return to the pot. Add the melon and shrimp and cook for another hour. Adjust the flavor with salt and pepper to taste. *8 servings*

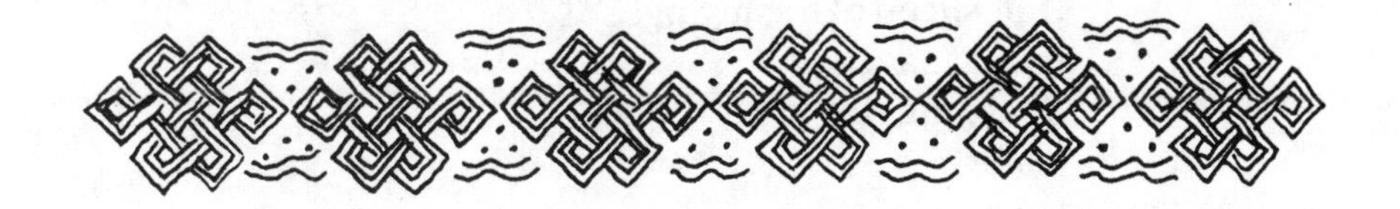

Corn and Crab Soup

6 C. fresh or prepared chicken stock
1 T. sesame oil
1 C. cooked crab meat
2 C. fresh or prepared corn kernels
1 T. plus 1 t. soy sauce
1 T. cornstarch dissolved in 3 T. cold water
3 spring onions, minced
1 T. cilantro leaves, minced
dash of hot sesame oil, to taste

In a non-reactive pot, combine the chicken stock, sesame oil, crab, corn, soy sauce, and cornstarch mixture. Bring to a boil, add the spring onions, and simmer for 5 minutes. Season with hot oil to taste and serve topped with cilantro leaves.

6 servings

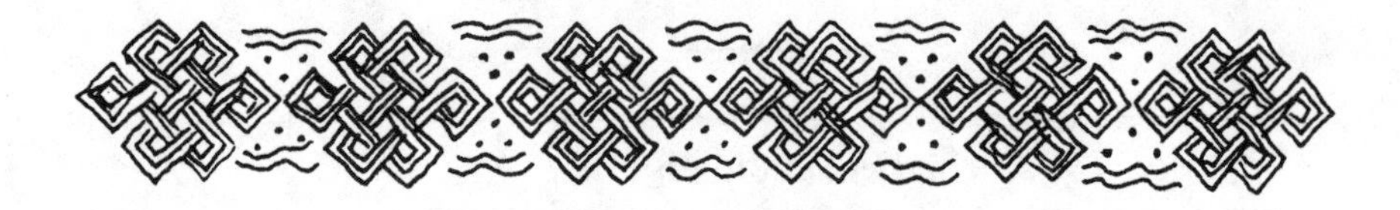

Beef and Oyster Sauce

1½	lb.	lean flank steak, sliced thin
1	t.	baking powder
1	t.	sugar
1	T.	cornstarch dissolved in 2 T. water
2	T.	soy sauce
4	T.	cooking oil
18		spring onions, cut into 2-inch pieces
18		thin slices of fresh ginger
2	t.	oyster sauce
2	T.	Shaoxing rice wine
1	t.	sugar
1	t.	sesame oil

Cut the beef slices into 2-inch strips. Mix together the baking powder, sugar, cornstarch mixture, and soy sauce in a shallow pan and marinate the beef for 1 hour or more. Heat the cooking oil in a *wok*. Saute the beef, ginger, and spring onions until done. Add the oyster sauce, wine, sugar, and sesame oil. Stir and serve hot.

6 servings

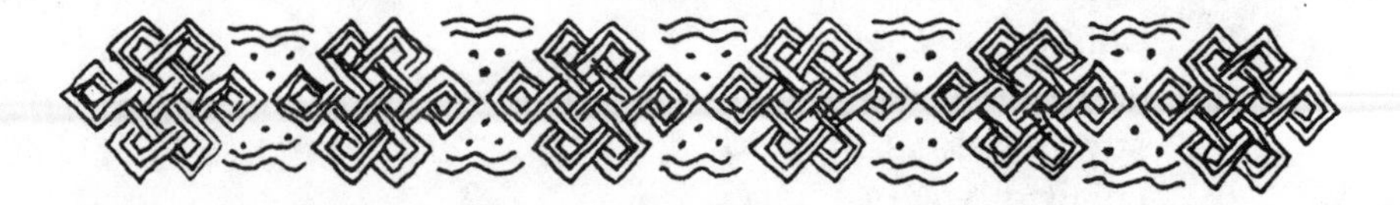

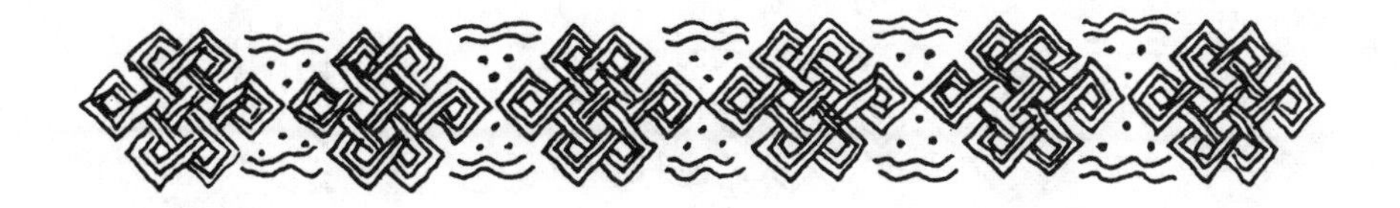

Autumn Pumpkin Rolls

2	lb.	pumpkin, peeled and diced
3	T.	cooking oil
2		leeks, cleaned and cut into matchsticks
12		slices of ginger, minced
6		dried black mushrooms, soaked, rinsed, and minced
1	T.	soy sauce
		ground white pepper to taste
1/4	C.	Shaoxing wine
12		spring roll wrappers
		flour paste (made by mixing 1 tablespoon instant flour with 2–3 tablespoons hot water)
		up to 1 C. cooking oil

Boil the pumpkin until tender, then drain and mash. Heat 3 tablespoons cooking oil in a *wok* or skillet. Brown the leeks, ginger, and mushrooms. Add the soy sauce, pepper to taste, and Shaoxing wine. Add the pumpkin and stir until well mixed. Divide the mixture into twelve portions. Place 1 portion on each wrapper and roll the wrappers into cylinders. Seal with flour paste. Fry in a clean skillet, using up to 1 cup of cooking oil. Serve hot. *6 servings*

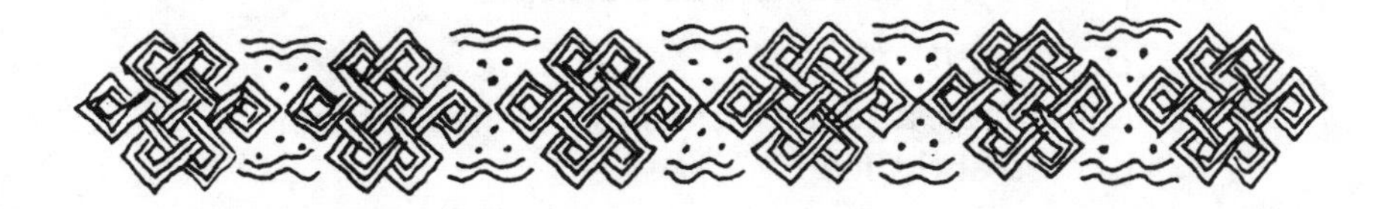

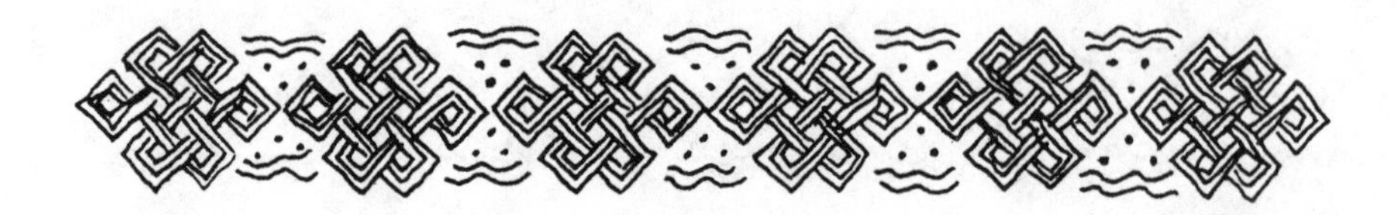

Pea Shoots with Seafood Sauce

2 T. cooking oil
3 slices of fresh ginger, minced
4 C. pea shoots
1 C. fish or chicken stock
1 C. cooked seafood (mix scallops, shrimp, etc., or just use one kind)
2 T. Shaoxing rice wine
2 t. sesame oil
1 egg white, lightly beaten

Heat the cooking oil in a *wok* or skillet over medium heat. Rinse the pea shoots and, with the water that clings to them, stir them into the heated *wok* or skillet. Stir until done, then remove and reserve. Add the stock to the *wok* and stir in the seafood. Add the wine and sesame oil and stir. Lightly beat the egg white and stir into the mixture. When thickened, pour over pea shoots and serve.

4 servings

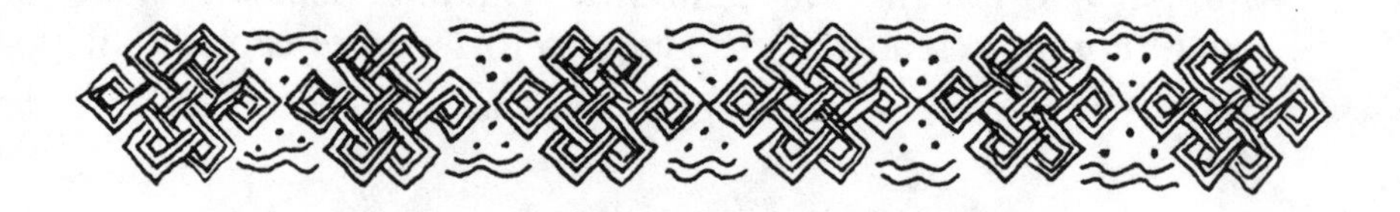

Stir-Fried Kohlrabi and Beef

3 T. cooking oil
3 kohlrabies, about 4 inches to 5 inches in diameter, peeled and sliced

6	cloves of garlic, peeled and sliced
3	slices of fresh ginger, minced
1 lb.	lean beef steak, sliced thin
2 T.	oyster sauce

Heat the oil in a *wok*. Stir fry the kohlrabi, then add garlic and ginger. Stir in the beef and stir fry until cooked. Add the oyster sauce, heat, and serve. *4 servings*

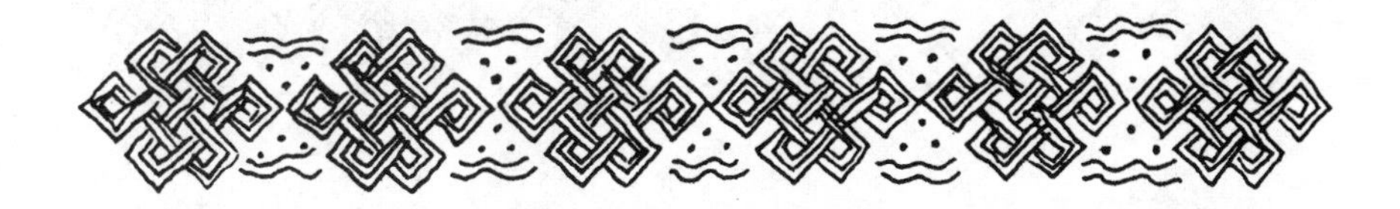

Sauteed Squid and Peppers

1 lb.	fresh squid
1 C.	self-rising flour
1 t.	baking powder
1/3 C.	water
2 T.	peanut oil
3 C. plus 1 T.	cooking oil
2 T.	cooking oil
1	large onion, peeled and cut into rings, then cut into 2-inch sections
1	red sweet pepper, seeded and cut into 2-inch squares
1	green sweet pepper, seeded and cut into 2-inch squares
1 T.	coarse salt
1 T.	five-spice powder

Wash and dry the squid and cut into 2-inch pieces. Mix together the flour, baking powder, water, and 2 tablespoons peanut oil to form a batter. Heat 3 cups of cooking oil in a *wok* or deep fryer, according to manufacturer's directions. Dip the squid in the batter and deep fry until golden brown and crisp, about 3 minutes.

Drain the squid on a paper towel and set aside. In a clean *wok* with 2 tablespoons cooking oil, saute the onion and peppers. Mix together the salt and spice powder. When cooked, stir in the squid and sprinkle with some of the salt mixture. Serve on a warm platter with the remaining salt mixture on the side.

4 servings

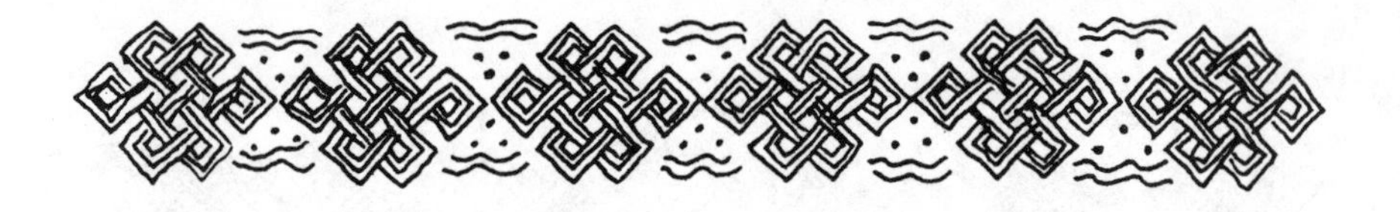

Spun Apples and Bananas

1	C.	all-purpose flour
1		egg, lightly beaten
½	C.	cold water
2		apples, peeled, cored, and cut into 2-inch pieces
2		bananas, peeled and cut into 2-inch slices
3	C.	peanut or safflower oil
1	C.	sugar
¼	C.	water
1	T.	cooking oil
1	T.	black sesame seeds
		large bowl of ice water

Place the flour in a large mixing bowl. Make a batter by beating in the egg and water. Lightly coat a serving platter with oil and set aside.

Place a bowl of ice water on the work table. In a *wok* or deep fryer, heat 3 cups of oil to 375° or according to manufacturer's directions. Heat the sugar, water, and 1 tablespoon oil in a skillet and boil until the sugar dissolves. Add the sesame seeds and leave on the lowest possible heat.

Dip the apple and banana pieces in the batter and deep fry until they are a light golden brown. With a slotted spoon, remove them from the oil and roll them in the sugar syrup. When they are coated, remove them with chopsticks or a slotted spoon and drop in the ice water. Retrieve them immediately and place them on the oiled serving platter. This dish takes a few tries to get right, but no matter how it looks, it usually tastes fine. *6 servings*

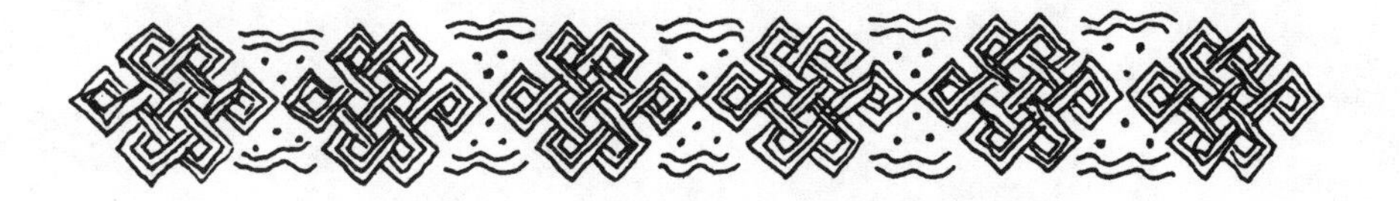

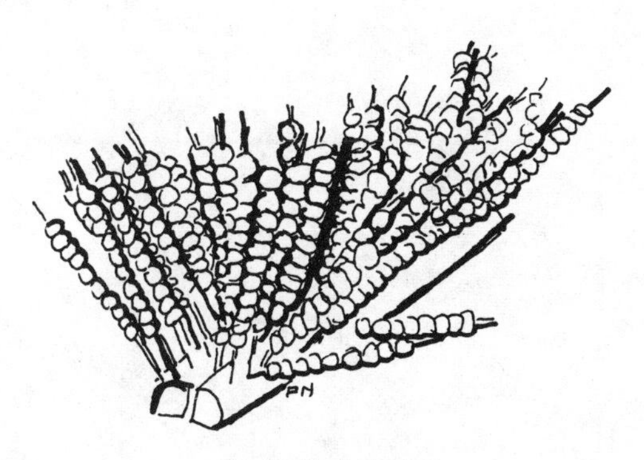

Candied Lady Apples

8

TAIPEI, TAIWAN

Sunday

It is 2:45 A.M. and I am eating fresh, sweet melon and drinking hot green tea. Both are delicious. It is a relaxing way to finish a meal of General Tso's Chicken, rice with crisp vegetables, and dry-cooked long beans.

The reason I am eating at this hour is because I am on a China Airlines jet flying to Taipei, where it is 2:45 tomorrow afternoon. Everyone has their own system for adjusting their internal clock. Mine is to ease into my approaching time zone with no subtlety at all. I get on the plane, set my watch for where I'm going, and do the best I can. Most of the time it works for me.

China Airlines makes it easy. The crew coordinates this off-hour meal as though everyone should have a banquet at this hour. We are handed hot towels before and after eating. After an equally delicious period of sleep, breakfast is served: *congee* with three pickles, cucumber, shredded pork, minced chicken, greens, a cold rolled omelet with fish, and a hot, sweet steamed roll. I accompany it with green tea. What a great way to wake up! The portions are huge and seconds are available. The plating is very pleasing—and there are chopsticks and a spoon on a rest.

I am very comfortable—even the headsets are user friendly, and the Western and Chinese musical selections are entertaining. From time to time the screen in front of us shows our route and other flight information on a map that is identified in Chinese and English. After various films we are served what the menu calls "lunch."

The first course is a smoked-salmon *hors d'oeuvre* tied with strips of seaweed, dressed with cracked pepper, and accompanied by eggs, caviar, beef, cucumber, and paté on field lettuce. On any other airline, this would have been the entire meal. It is followed by poached fish in a mild white sauce with carrots and peas. Dessert is a fresh fruit plate: pineapple, papaya, strawberry, and starfruit. For a while I drift in and out of sleep.

Over the Sea of Hokosai I start to feel elated, eager, and responsive. I take out my drawing paper and pen and start to draw. The sun is coming up, somehow behind us; to the left, the clouds are whitening and thickening until I cannot see through them.

As we descend, there are fields and fields of rice, and in the place of about every tenth field is a rectangular pond used both for irrigation and fish farming. Along the road to Taipei from the airport the fields are colored like a child's drawing of grass using the brightest crayon in the box, an exuberant late-spring green. They exude the energy of Kansas wheat fields. There are factories and fields of rice. . . an oil refinery and fields of rice. . . suburban and semi-urban communities everywhere interspersed with gardens of tufted rice. I think I must be wrong, that this is simply wild grass gone amok, but the limo driver says, "Of course it's rice."

No wonder most Taiwanese like New York. It is morning rush hour and we are crawling along past road-level construction and under an elevated freeway being built. We continue beside piggy-back flat beds, Mercedes, and thousands of mopeds and motor scooters. Some people wear helmets, but most are without, including a young mother with two small children. I can't keep my eyes from them until they turn off. The radio station we are listening to broadcasts in Chinese and English, and at this hour it plays reggae and soft rock between news and traffic updates. The large number of scooters, arcaded buildings, and narrow-angled streets radiating from wide avenues make the city look alive and exciting.

The Lai Lai Sheraton is a model of efficiency; it is clear that my every need will be met as planned or with an equally comforting alternative.

After a quick wash and change, I meet representatives from the Taiwan Tourism Bureau in the lobby at 10:30. They are charming and generous with their time and information. We are on our way to meet Teresa Lin, the consultant for the Chinese Gourmet Association. We talk first about her work as the food consultant for "Eat, Drink, Man, Woman," Ang Lee's new movie about food, family life, tradition, and breaking free. I told her that no one I knew could take their eyes from the food long enough to follow the film's plot and were constantly asking, "What happened? What did she say?" Not only did Teresa style most of the food shots, but she also came up with some of the dishes, such as the oversized "beggar's chicken" that the father in the movie smashes quite a bit harder than necessary to free the tender roasted bird from its hard-baked shell. She was also the one who put together the 750 kilos of food for the opening-night party at Cannes, and more recently, she brought six chefs to Los Angeles to give a banquet for 1,000 people to promote "Eat, Drink, Man, Woman" for an Oscar.

Teresa's father cooked not professionally, but very well. She studied languages at Fujien Catholic University, took some courses in design and nutrition, put them together, and became a food designer. She is also called in as a consultant on many social programs, such as the current one in Taipei that trains people in prison to cook, improving the prison food as well as the prisoners' morale and job opportunities upon release.

Teresa is exuberant and will pick me up at 8:30 the following morning to go to the food market, after which we will meet the others at an agreed-upon *dim sum* restaurant. She recommends that for a night-time snack I go to the *dan dan* noodle parlor at the "City of Cathay." One of my new acquaintances says, "Of course. We will go tonight." He will pick me up at 4:00, and we will go first to the deputy director general of the Tourism Bureau.

The Chung-Hsiao Restaurant is in a busy downtown alley. It has several branches and sells packaged food as well. One way to start lunch is with a cold plate of spiced kelp, bean curd, and tea eggs, accompanied by *sha ping*, small baked buns covered in sesame seeds and filled with soy-sauced mutton. The *ching kung* noodles are served in a tasty broth with local gourds, dried mushrooms, lily flower buds, mushrooms, and pork. It is the assortment of sweet cakes and snacks that one finds at Chung Hsiao that are a learning experience. Among the ones I liked were *kuei hua* cake (made of glutinous rice flour, stuffed with sweetened bean paste, steamed, and served cold with a syrup of sugar and osmanthus), sliced lotus root, with its canals filled with glutinous rice and boiled in aromatic syrup, haw jelly cake (much like guava paste), and a sweetened violet rice cake that is said to encourage longevity. Other "lucky" cakes are a five-layer square cake, a single-layer cake of glutinous rice, and another of red bean paste, violet rice, sesame paste, and mashed jujubes. Another is the elephant's trunk cake: glutinous rice stuffed with mashed jujubes and osmanthus, rolled in sesame seeds, and shaped like an elephant's trunk. Also there are, of course, the traditional sweet broths and tea made from varieties of nuts, seeds, or beans.

It is now 2:00. I haven't slept in a bed for three nights, but I feel terrific. Back at the hotel, I think about napping, but instead go up to the pool and health club. I go to the women's sauna room, where hand-held showers have terrific water pressure to scrub at tired skin, then into a hot tub followed by an immersion in cold water and a brief sauna. After an hour's rest, I am downstairs at 4:00.

The deputy director of the Bureau of Tourism is a graduate of the University of Michigan, where he studied, among other things, forestry, and is a fierce environmentalist. Highly regarded as the "father of Taiwan's national parks," he promotes ecotourism and encourages the exploration of the geological and biological diversity of the island. He does not want to talk about himself, but instead talks about the food festival that has occurred in Taipei every year since 1990. The organizers invite chefs from all parts of China to participate and demonstrate Chinese cooking, from the court and mansion style to the home and daily fare of the general population. The presentation varies from intricate food carving to steamed fresh vegetables that are so bright and crisp they look like food sculpture.

Dinner is at Tien Hsiang Lo, which is arguably the best traditional Hangzhou (Hang Chow) or West Lake food in Taiwan. Hangzhou is the capital of Zhejiang province. At the time of Marco Polo's visit, it had a population of 1 million. Abundant rice fields and waterways have for centuries marked the area as a center for fish and rice. West Lake has been rendered by many artists and has traditionally been a gathering place for people with a love of nature, art, and poetry. It is also famous for *lungjing* or "Dragon Well" tea.

We are met by Angela Tsai, assistant to Stanley Yen, the president of the Ritz Hotel, and Lily Liang, the director of public relations. Most of the hotel is in the art deco style, but we enter the restaurant as though through a small Chinese courtyard. It is a room with about twenty-five tables set with white cloths, flowers, and the silver-plated spoon and chopsticks stands used in most upscale places.

We start with an array of cold appetizers including drunken chicken, preserved duck, pickled radish, and smoked fish (smoked over brown sugar, rice, and tea leaves). Jason Ong, the director of food and beverages, comes by to explain the process as well as how the cold dishes are prepared without preservatives in a slow, traditional way. He also explains that the fish balls in the soup we are about to eat have to be made by hand. The ground fish is so delicate that the touch of the chef's hands is what heats the mixture just enough to hold it together. The water lily soup with fish balls is something you would like to be able to send out for on a winter's night. The slivers of water lily leaves have a taste almost like sweet seaweed. They also slightly thicken the soup without any additives, and a touch of ginger adds to the aroma. The West Lake fish is served with cucumbers and edible flowers, a modern touch. Dessert has the same name it always does: sweet glutinous rice balls. I would never order that, would you? But they are good, two small rice balls in a thin sauce of pureed pineapple and banana almost like a floating island. During our meal we drink *lon ching cha*, as our cups are frequently refilled and reheated. I cannot remember a "working" meal where I ate so much of everything.

I learn more about Hangzhou (Hang Chow) cooking. The West Lake has been immortalized in paintings and poetry as a beautiful natural spot. About 1000 A.D. the Widow Song and her son lived there. When the son was ill, she fed him with fish stock thickened with fish bones and lotus, which are still used as a natural thickener by purists today.

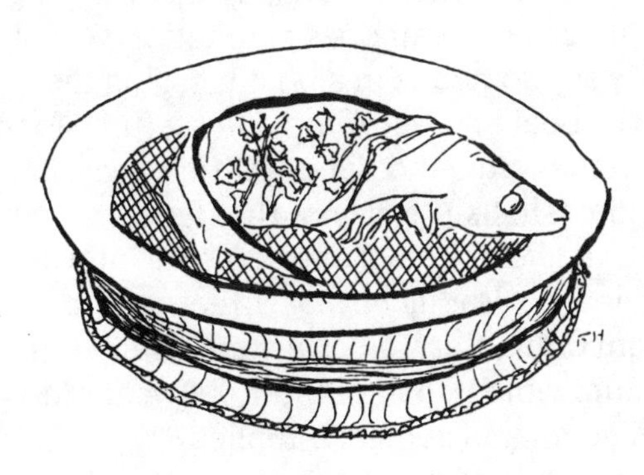

West Lake Fish

Then the Widow Song prepared the fish for him and doused it with wine, vinegar, and sugar. Her brother-in-law came by and tasted it. He was so enthusiastic that he encouraged her to open a restaurant near the lake. It was successful, and when the emperor heard of these fabulous dishes, he sent for her. But not wishing to obey a despot, the widow ran off, some say with her brother-in-law. This is a popular Chinese culinary story that serves not only as an origin for some recipes, but as a reminder that women chefs and restaurateurs are still few and far between.

After dinner, we drive through a still-busy city. It is almost 8:00 and many places are open; there are people everywhere. As we go through the streets, it appears that one of the reasons the food in Taipei is generally so good is that there are many styles of eating places at many price levels, allowing people with a diversity of employment to eat well. For some reason, the biggest Western surprise for me is the presence of 7–11 stores. There are, of course, the ubiquitous McDonald's, Burger Kings (and the local competition, Burger Queen), and a Japanese company called Mos Burger that makes a hamburger between two rice patties. There are local ice creams and sorbets, but Häagen Daz and Baskin Robbins are still visible.

On to the "City of Cathay," which is a reconstruction of an old-time generic Chinese village with handicrafts and lots of food stalls. We wander about a bit, enjoying young students of the performing arts who are doing the dragon dance and other traditional mime and dance stories. My favorite, because of the costumes, is a story about an old man carrying a young girl (acted by one performer with a complicated costume) away from her lover, a guy with a big papier-mâché head. In the next scene, a man does acrobatics with his paddle while he rows, then we see someone in a boat crossing the water. Each person, as well as the boat and water, are one costume for one performer. Then a man is in the water and dances with a beautiful clam. Incredible sequinned clamshells the size of the dancer's body are attached to her arms so that she can envelope someone at will.

We cannot leave without having street-stall *dan dan* noodles. I can't believe I am doing this. I not only eat some of the noodles and, with some encouragement, half of the 1,000-year old egg, but sip the broth. I say it is good, and someone replies, "When you are hungry, it is delicious." We look at each other and laugh.

I prove that I have a sense of humor, because next we go a few paces down to a tea house. We are served tea, which comes with an assortment of tiny assorted sweets; the gelatin ones are the best. Yes, I did try them. This is a local comedy club, and on stage is a young man with an earring dressed in an old-style Mandarin robe. The story he is telling is about language and dialects, and he does a comic dialogue of a father-son conversation that ultimately turns into a song. He is hilarious and we end the evening in laughter.

Monday

It is a beautiful morning, rather like the first clear day at the end of summer when there is no humidity in the air. Wide awake, I go out for a walk around the block. School children of all ages wear backpacks, walking and buying the fried eggs or grilled cheese sandwiches being freshly made by the street vendors on the same iron grills they will use later in the day to make spring roll skins.

I want to get to the National Palace Museum at 10:00. I take a cab alone, passing first through urban activity, then along tree-lined avenues and past more island-like streets, palm trees, simpler store fronts, women in cotton dresses, and houses in the hills. We drive up a curved road lined with tapered yew trees; when we reach the museum, we are properly impressed. It is four times as large as I expected. Its art and artifacts are exquisite, and I also take the time to learn a little history.

Located in the Pacific Ocean, with the Philippines 210 miles (350 kilometers) to the south and Japan 650 miles (1,000 kilometers) to the north, Taiwan is separated from Fujian province by ninety-five miles (160 kilometers) across the Strait of Taiwan. With its beautiful beaches and green central mountains, Taiwan has been populated for thousands of years. Though it is subject to monsoons, typhoons, and an average rainfall of one hundred inches a year, the island has given shelter to seafarers from near and far throughout its history.

Though there are various theories about the origins of the indigenous people, the migration of Chinese groups is thought to have begun with the Hakka around 1000 C.E. and the next large wave of settlers from Fujian, who arrived at the fall of the Ming Dynasty in 1644

C.E. Even at that time there was trade not only in deer hides but in powdered deer horn, which was thought to be an aphrodisiac. The Chinese named the island Taiwan. At about the same time, Portuguese navigators named it "*Ilha Formosa*," or "Beautiful Island," but it was the Dutch who first claimed it as a base for their Asian trade.

Both Spain and Japan tried to establish ports there, but the Dutch drove them out. They in turn were driven out by the Ming naval force, which made the island a part of Fujian province. By the nineteenth century, the West started showing interest in the island again, and the U.S. even considered buying it. By the end of the Sino-Japanese War of 1895, Taiwan came under Japanese rule through the Treaty of Shimonoscki.

The main food of the island was fish and seafood in great variety. Rice and tea were cultivated and fruit and vegetables were abundant. Taiwanese cuisine makes full use of these ingredients in dishes that are most frequently sauteed or steamed and that show a preference for fresh rather than preserved ingredients. The food styles of the various nations involved in Taiwan's history have influenced some dishes, but none so much as Japan. This influence is still apparent.

At the end of the Second World War in 1945, the island was returned to the Chinese people. In 1949, when the People's Republic of China was established in Beijing, the Kuomingtang, under the leadership of Generalissimo Chiang Kaishek, spearheaded the settlement of an estimated 2 million people in Taiwan and declared Taipei the provisional capital of the Republic of China. Since they came from all parts of China, they brought with them the cooks and cooking styles of many regions. Now, in Taiwan as in most major Chinese cities, you can get authentic food in the manner of diverse culinary traditions, and with open exchanges there is less of a systematic classification and a great deal of overlapping.

After four decades, martial law in Taiwan was lifted and in 1988 Lee Teng-hui became the first president of Taiwan who was not a member of the Kuomingtang. The election presaged a modern era of social and political mobility.

Although I am reluctant to leave the museum, I must get back for a meeting with Mary Yang, a restaurateur and designer and the owner and executive chef at Fu Yuen.

Located on a narrow alley, Fu Yuen's building would invite picture-taking if one didn't know it was a restaurant. And, if you didn't know this housed one of the best restaurants in Asia, there is no sign or symbol indicating that it is open to the public.

In 1988 Mary Yang bought the land where the restaurant is located; it took three years to build. After working thirteen years as the chef in a mansion, Ms. Yang knew exactly what she wanted—an expression of the timelessness of Chinese architecture. It was designed consciously and deliberately to express aesthetic integrity and seriousness. Ms. Yang doesn't care about its being a "fun" place—but a pleasurable place, now that's another thing.

The restaurant has ten private rooms, for the most part designed like a scholar's studio, each with its own antechamber furnished in antiques of museum quality. One circular *cloisonné* top is larger and more detailed than any other I have seen. Wood is used for the ribs in the domed ceilings that are hung with elaborate lanterns. Each large room is different from the others; some have the ribs steamed and curved as the ribs of a ship, while others have ribs that are angled and intricately stepped up to a peak. Wood screenwork is everywhere, and the woodwork of the floors is as smooth as the deck of a ship. Most of the walls are hand-rubbed plaster and the tables, chairs, and side pieces are well selected. But it is the selection of art on the walls that is breathtaking. Carefully framed calligraphy from all periods, including a piece by the last emperor's brother Pu Jie, hang on the walls. Of course, there are family and corporate special banquet celebrations held here, but this is also a place where governments invite other governments to eat.

Each large room has its own prep and clean-up kitchen, and there is a proper kitchen on every other floor, with the largest on the bottom floor. Even the staff dining room has calligraphy framed on the walls and handsome tables and chairs. Stainless steel is everywhere, and although Ms. Yang calls the restaurant her stage, it seems somehow more complex than that. Every detail reflects her appreciation and knowledge of culture.

We tour the bathrooms, matte-finished pale marble on most floors and partially up the walls, carved wooden doors, small watercolors, and marble sink counters. The lights and mirrors would make anyone pleased with their appearance. There are also a few intimate rooms that accommodate four to eight people; they are also that well appointed. We are going to eat in the open dining room, which has ten tables, each seating four to six. Most of them are occupied. As we start to eat, Mary Yang aerates the wine in each glass. She is rushing a bit, she says, because she is taking a management course and must be at school by 2:30.

Her detractors say she has gone too far. I cannot believe they would say this after eating the sauteed duck liver in wine, oyster sauce, and honey while sipping a Bordeaux that has been carefully aerated. Other dishes include jellyfish wrapped in vegetable leaves; squid and leek bundles; fried, stuffed bamboo shoots served with slices of roast goose, duck, and cucumber; and *dofu* in the shape of small fish with pea pods cut to look like tails and fins and accompanied by crabmeat sauce. The dessert is a traditional molded almond gel with sliced kiwi, honeydew, starfruit, and fruit sauce.

The service is attentive and all the plates are carefully positioned to show off their best appearance.

Back at the Lai Lai Sheraton, I meet with Jane Lu and Executive Chef Chang Hwa Chou, who is in charge of the food here and also the food consultant for China Airlines. He is so calm and good natured it is hard to believe that he is "on call" all the time. There are several Chinese restaurants at the Lai Lai in addition to those of an international variety. Each restaurant has its own kitchen and the chef visits them daily in the morning and evening. In addition to all the things "being in charge" means, he also keeps up to date with new trends and is an important person at the annual T'aipei Chinese Food Festival.

Chang Hwa Chou's style is very uncluttered and his presentation is very restrained and elegant. Used to designing menus for travelers from Asia and the West, his food is a very good introduction for people who may at first be overwhelmed by the large varieties of unknown morsels in many traditional Taiwanese dishes. His two most popular appetizers are almond fried shrimp and fried-chicken spring roll.

One of the specialties he demonstrates is *wok* cooking, and his light touch with oil and the intense flavor of his dishes in taste are the work of a virtuoso. The emphasis is on fish and very fresh leafy vegetables with shallots, ginger, and garlic or simply spring onions and ginger. Color and nutritional value are important to him. For a casual meal he might serve four or five dishes at the same time, but not all mixed together as some Western restaurants might. We talk about traditional service for longer meals: moving from light dishes to heavy and then back to light. A menu he likes might include a cold-cut platter with smoked and pickled selections, sauteed seafood, braised shark's fin soup, a spicy mutton dish, steamed fish, and sauteed mixed vegetables. Next would come *yu won tang* (a broth soup with bamboo and fishballs made with an equal amount of ground fish and squid for texture, mixed with egg white, minced ginger and spring onion, and held together by a bit of lard). The soup is served with bits of tomato and spinach to add some color. Two desserts, both dumplings, one savory and one sweet, and then fruit in season would be served.

We tour the hotel food-service areas and both the Hunan Garden and Happy Garden Restaurants. The large staff works as though a choreographer were in charge. The immaculate modern kitchens are busy and productive. The cooking utensils vary slightly from ones that would be recognized from history; others are cutting edge. We are politely ignored, smiled at, or greeted warmly—a sure sign of the comfort level at the "back of the house." In part Chang Hwa Chou is so relaxed because his father was a pastry chef, and he grew up with a sense of professionalism, although nothing could have compared to the scale of his current stewardship. More importantly, I think he keeps a sense of balance and humor by jogging and taking long mountain walks in the beautiful countryside.

Tuesday

I meet Teresa Lin as planned. Our first stop is the East Market. There is a large selection of vegetables, fruit, fish, dried beans, and even packaged food. We go to the family-run stall of a *dofu* maker. The aroma of the *dofu* settling in large wooden tubs is so good it makes me hungry. I am not the only one, and we each eat large bowls. I can't quite believe I am eating slightly warm *dofu*, with some liquid still in it, and it tastes better than *créme caramel*. Talk about comfort food! I watch as the *dofu* is drained, pressed to various thicknesses, and shaped on hand-made wooden frames and molds.

Next we wander among the seafood stalls: live shrimp, crabs, and fish, dried and soaked cuttlefish, and soaking sea slugs or sea cucumbers (often called, even in Asia, *bêche-de-mer*) that become seven times larger wet than when they are dry. These should only be bought from reliable vendors; they are not tasty if they have soaked too long.

Suddenly there is a great rumble and the floor shifts. This earthquake, it turns out, has registered 5.6 on the Richter scale. Teresa and I instinctively move away from under a large fan that has strings attached to keep the flies from the food. Everything and everyone becomes still, then we shrug and continue as we were three seconds earlier. It is like the cliché shot in a movie when the frame is frozen for the flicker of an eye, then moves, as if to pursue that image further would be too disruptive of the story at hand. We continue our walk and try to name all the leaves we see in both Chinese and English. Cabbages, cresses, spinaches, peas, sprouts, shoots, mushrooms, roots, beans, snake squashes, and bottle gourds are in abundance. We see both the "good heart" plant and the "empty heart" vegetable, old ginger with the tough skin we are familiar with, and young ginger with smooth, pale paper-thin skin and pink tips.

We stop also at the South Gate Market where, in addition to stalls of fruit and vegetables, there are large varieties of prepared food—"take out." The list of items available is so long that one could shop here every day for a year and not repeat the same dinner.

Rita Wong and Robin Lin are the directors of the Foundation of Chinese Dietary Culture. They graciously offer me cassia tea, which is surprisingly good, and tell me about their work. Anyone with a professional or serious interest in the subject may join the foundation. It offers not only an extensive library of books and periodicals, but also has audio and video tapes as well as on-line computer services. There are regular meetings, classes, and seminars, and notes from these events are available as well. Started in 1987, the foundation is quickly becoming a vast repository of information.

I go to the Din Tai Fung Restaurant for lunch and then, as it turns out, both dinner and a midnight supper. While in college twenty years ago, Yang Chi Hua, an authentic polymath and the restaurant's present owner and executive chef, saw the then chef make a kind of dumpling that fascinated him. He got a job working there with the chef and continued on in school. They used to send the owner away to play *mah jong* so that Yang Chi Hua could practice making the dumplings until they were perfect.

Yang Chi Hua is friendly, smiling, and generous with his time, although the place is so busy that the wait staff uses walkie-talkies. Guests enter this three-story, hundred-table restaurant through the kitchen where everything is made.

When asked how the dumplings are made, Yang Chi Hua is happy to say that the dumpling skins are made from a yeast dough, each day's batch being produced from the starter left from the previous day's batch. They are simply made from the starter mixed with bread flour and water and then filled. (As an example, one version is filled with one-third crabmeat, two-thirds pork, and seasoned with ginger and spring onions.)

The dumplings filled with soup are hard to describe; they are partially filled with a chicken and jellied *consommé* mixture that turns to liquid when they have been cooked. They are accompanied by pickled cabbage, pickled seaweed, and sauces of vinegar, shredded ginger, and hot pepper. The server pours the tea, holding the kettle at least a meter above the smallish teacup, a signature gesture.

We talk and when I say I have eaten a lifetime of dumplings and never tasted anything with the same layering of tastes and textures, he explains that a couple of chefs from another country wanted to pay him for permission to come and work with him for a week. He told them he couldn't possibly charge them because they wouldn't learn to make the dumplings in so short a time. They came, stayed a week, and didn't.

There are various soups; the two I sampled were the black chicken, which was wonderful, and the hot-and-sour soup, which had pork strips, blood pudding, and bamboo shoots. They may call this simply hot-and-sour soup, but that gives an image of the ubiquitous sour, slimy stuff we get at most places; this has a dozen distinct flavors. Yang Chi Hua says it is easy—just use the best ingredients and cook them well. (It is the same advice Paul Bocuse gives.)

It is now evening, and I am committed to going to Ting Tai Feng because, in a very generous way, Yang Chi Hua has asked me to join a group of his painter friends who meet every Wednesday at 8:00 to paint and bring in the paintings they are working on for critique by a master who also paints during this time.

I politely refuse at first, but the invitation sounds so sincere and the food so delicious, that I finally say yes and show up at 7:30. The restaurant is filled and everyone is working or eating. Yang Chi Hua is a born restaurateur; he shows me the menu, but orders for me, of course suggesting local beer. He joins me briefly and we chat. As I guessed, his English is much better than he lets on. The scene is marvelous—everyone has a walkie-talkie and the tea is poured from a meter above the cups. Dumplings and small dishes are never mixed on a steamer; each dish is served separately. Once again, I can't believe how much I am eating.

This place also makes more of a low-key, high-fashion statement than any place in New York, even though the tables are without tablecloths and you enter through the kitchen. Most people seemed to be Taiwanese and regulars, but there are also lots of travelers and many languages being spoken. One of the three Chinese women at the next table takes out a dictionary at the same time I do, so we both laugh. Originally from San Francisco, she has been here one year and is working for an English-language paper and improving her Chinese. Her aunts are from San Francisco and Vancouver and are visiting and having fun. Making the universal "ssh" sign, I pass my extra dumplings to them as they say they have waited eagerly to eat here since they first heard of it.

A little after 8:30 P.M., we go into the little room where we had the lunch meeting. The painting master and two of the students are unrolling paintings of the same scene. The master proceeds to correct the work in each painting. I practice holding the brush and making strokes. Embarrassed by my clumsiness, I show them my slides and resume, saying at least I am a member of the club.

They are very supportive and give me a brush and paper to start emulating the painting. I am less than successful. The ranges of pale gray to dense black, the thin lines, and the washes flowing from the brushes of the people around me demonstrate painting. From the same brush come both fine lines and bold. I made a few attempts at the scene, to some laughter and some encouragement. Finally I came up with an almost acceptable waterfall in the midst of some laughable rocks, then some decent vegetables that are in the right style and technique. There are six artists who speak from none to good English. We communicate just fine. The master gives me an ink drawing; one artist gives me a brush and another some paper. It becomes time to go, but one of the men suggests we first go upstairs for a snack, as part of the weekly routine. I barely believe the table that greets us: salmon *sashimi*, spicy eggplant with fish flavor, melon soup, pickles, and *liang* fish-head soup (large fish heads, bean noodles, and fried *dofu*) brewing on a gas burner in the middle of the table. Then the traditional cheers go up and there is armagnac followed by cognac. It seems this group is together because.of *tai chi*. I ask how often they practice; "everyday" is the answer.

Chef Chang Hwa Chou of the Lai Lai Sheraton in T'aipei has offered the following dishes with great success. Any of these are perfect appetizers for a party or would make a very good lunch for four people.

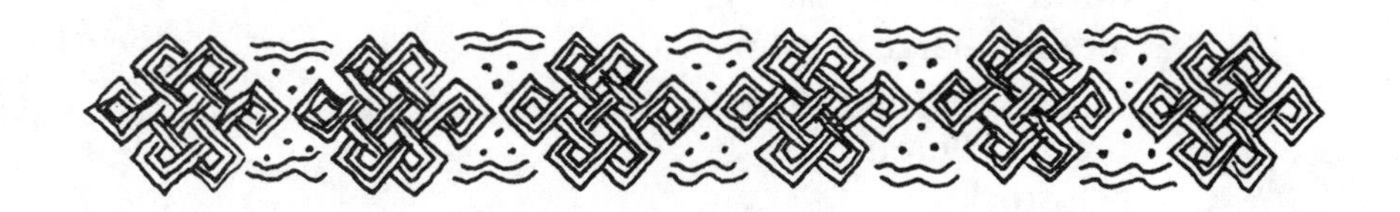

Almond Fried Shrimp

8	large shrimp
1	pinch of salt
1/4 t.	ground white pepper
2 t.	cornstarch dissolved in 2 T. cold water
2	eggs
2 T.	water
3/4 C.	flour
1 C.	slivered almonds
4 C.	oil for deep frying (or, if using a deep fryer, follow manufacturer's directions)
2	tomatoes for garnish

Shell the shrimp and devein. Mix together the salt, pepper, and cornstarch mixture. Soak the shrimp in the seasoning mixture, first on one side, then the other for a total of 10 minutes. Beat the eggs and water in a shallow bowl. Dip the shrimp in the flour, then in the beaten-egg mixture, and then in the slivered al-

monds. Fry in hot fat until golden brown, about 4 minutes. Drain and serve on a platter with tomatoes cut into decorative shapes as garnish.
4 servings

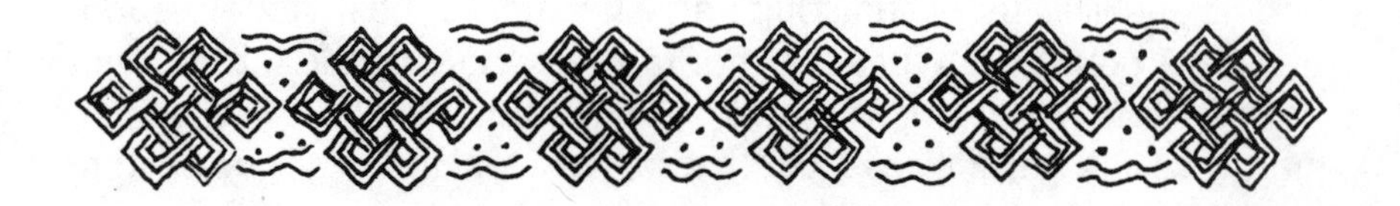

Steamed Sea Scallop Rolls

8		dried scallops (*conpoy*)
8		medium-large shrimp
		salt and pepper to taste
8		broccoli florets
1/2	C.	fish stock
2	t.	cornstarch dissolved in 2 T. cold water
1		egg, beaten
		lemon slices as garnish
2	T.	parsley for garnish, minced

Steam the dried scallops for 2 hours. Remove the shrimp's shell and devein. Make small cuts on the backs of the shrimp so that they do not curl. Boil the broccoli. Salt and pepper the shrimp, fold them around the scallops, and steam them over high heat for 7 minutes. Heat the fish stock and thicken it with cornstarch. Stir in the beaten egg until it is cooked through. Place the broccoli and the shrimp and scallops alternately on a plate. Drizzle fish stock over all and garnish with the lemon slices and parsley.
4 servings

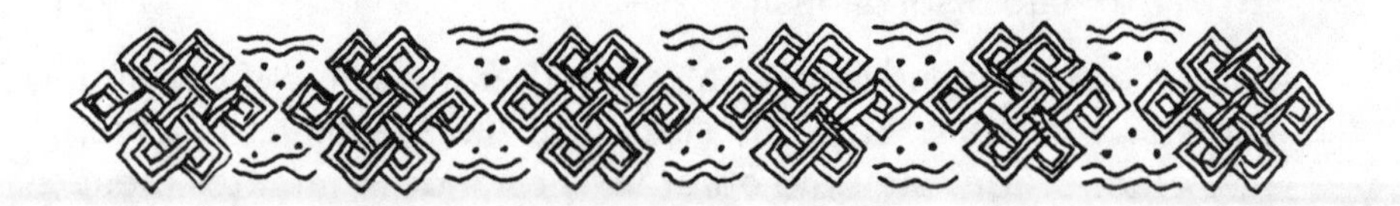

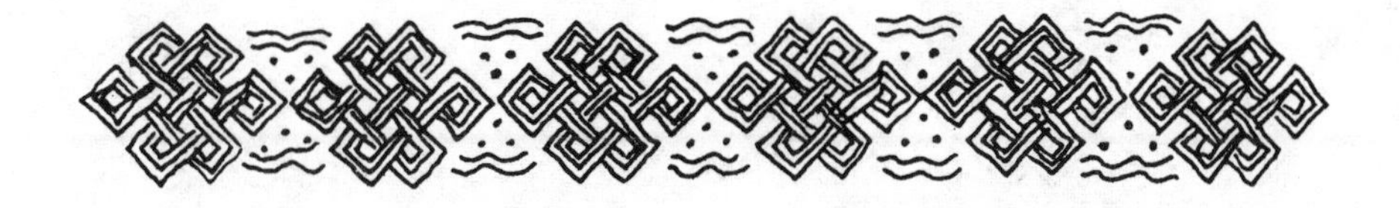

Fried-Chicken Spring Rolls

4		boneless chicken thighs, skin removed
½	C.	white button mushrooms
1	C.	bamboo shoots cut in pieces
¼	C.	preserved pickled vegetables
½	t.	powdered coriander seed
1	t.	sugar
1	t.	cornstarch
12		sheets of glutinous-rice spring wrappers
3	C.	oil for deep frying (or if using a deep fryer, follow manufacturer's instructions)

Julienne the chicken, mushrooms, and bamboo shoots. Mix with the seasoning and cornstarch and wrap in spring wrappers to form cylinders 1 inch in diameter and 4 inches long. Deep fry until golden brown. *6 servings*

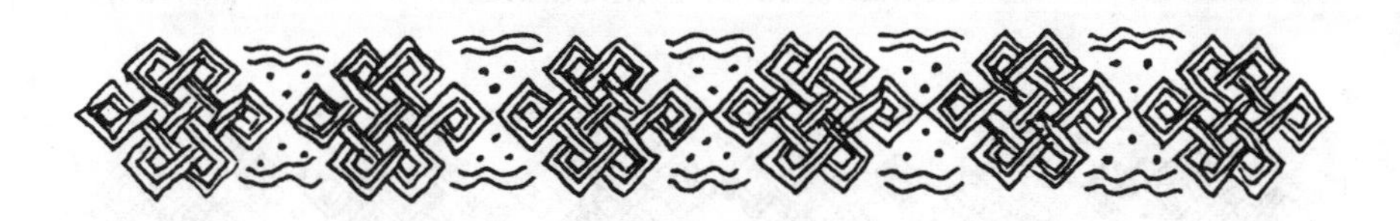

The following two recipes are from Chef Chiu of the Tien Hsiang Lo Restaurant at the Ritz Hotel in Taipei.

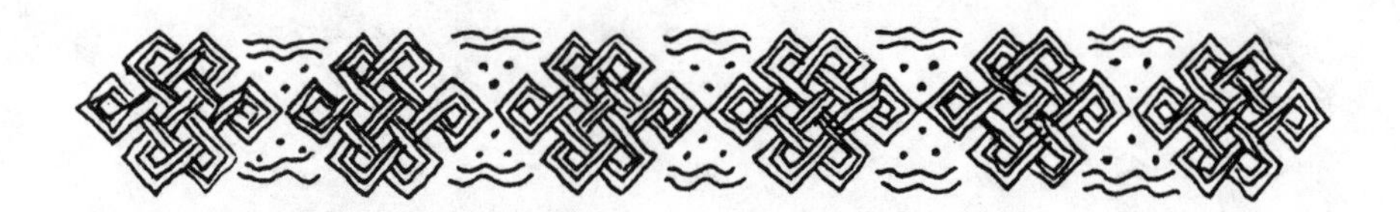

Braised Sponge Gourd (Peng Hua) with Fresh Bamboo Shoots

2	long sponge gourds, approximately 1 lb. each (Note: This gourd is really a zucchini-shaped melon and is often found at local markets with its blossom still attached.)
4 oz.	fresh bamboo shoots
2 T.	cooking oil
1 T.	oyster sauce
	salt to taste
1 T.	cornstarch dissolved in 3 T. of cold water

Peel, seed, and slice the sponge gourds. Scrape the bamboo shoots and slice. Heat the oil in a *wok* and add oyster sauce and salt to taste. Add the gourd and sliced bamboo shoots and cook until soft. Add the cornstarch mixture and stir until blended. Place on a warm dish and serve immediately. *4 servings*

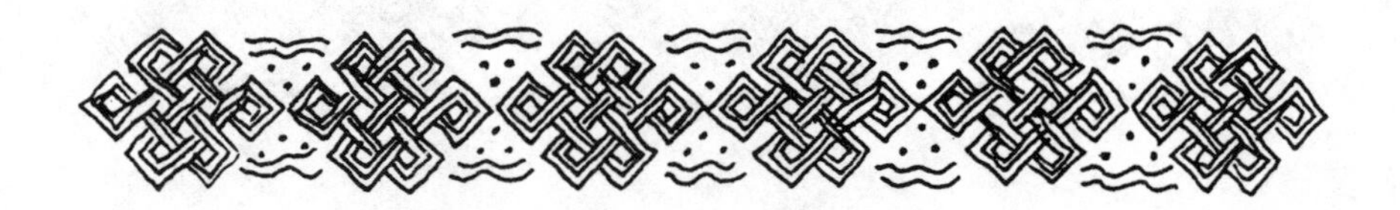

West Lake Fish Fillets

1½ lb.	grass fish fillets, cut in 6 pieces
1 T.	fresh ginger, minced
1 T.	Chinkiang vinegar
2 T.	soy sauce
2 T.	sugar

1 T.	sesame oil
2 T.	Shaoxing wine
2 t.	cornstarch dissolved in 2 T. cold water

Place enough water in a *wok* to cook the fish. Bring the water to a boil and gently simmer the fish for 3 minutes. Gently remove the fish, drain, and place on a warm platter. Pour the water out of the *wok* and return 1 cup of water to the *wok* and bring to a boil. Add the ginger, vinegar, soy sauce, sugar, and oil. Stir until sauce boils, then add the wine. Add the cornstarch mixture and stir until blended. Pour the hot sauce over the fish and serve immediately. *4 servings*

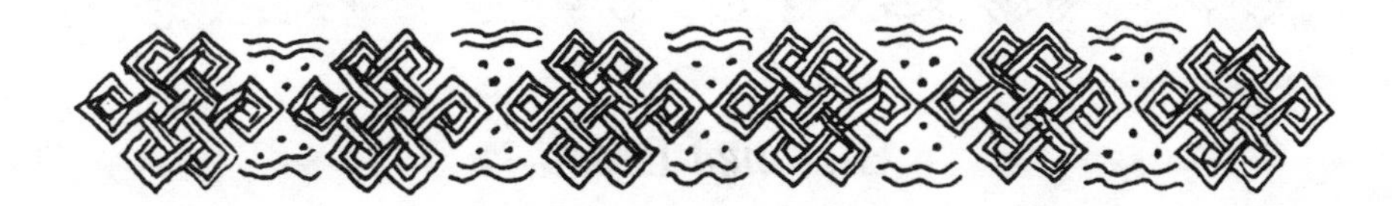

Teresa Lin has generously supplied the following recipes:

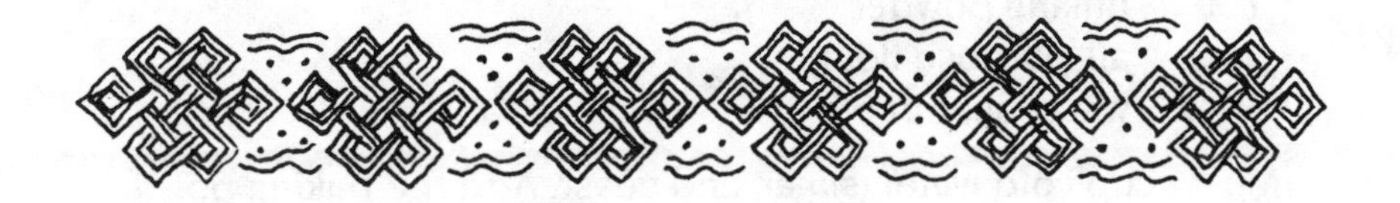

Baked Ham with Syrup

2 lb.	Chinese ham in one piece (Virginia ham may be substituted)
1 C.	Chinese sugar or brown sugar
1 C.	candied lotus seeds
12	pieces steamed bread

Soak the ham in hot water for ½ hour, then clean it with a brush. Place the ham in a bowl inside a steamer, cover with water, and steam for 1 hour. When the ham cools, discard the skin and cut into 1-inch x 2⅛-inch pieces. Put the ham into a clean bowl inside the steamer, and add 3 tablespoons of the sugar and ½ cup water. Steam for 1 hour. Drain, return to the bowl with another 3 tablespoons of sugar and ½ cup water, and steam for ½ hour. Drain the ham, rinse the bowl, and place the ham, candied lotus seeds, remaining sugar, and ½ cup water in it and steam for 20 minutes. Place on a warm plate and serve with steamed bread.

6 servings

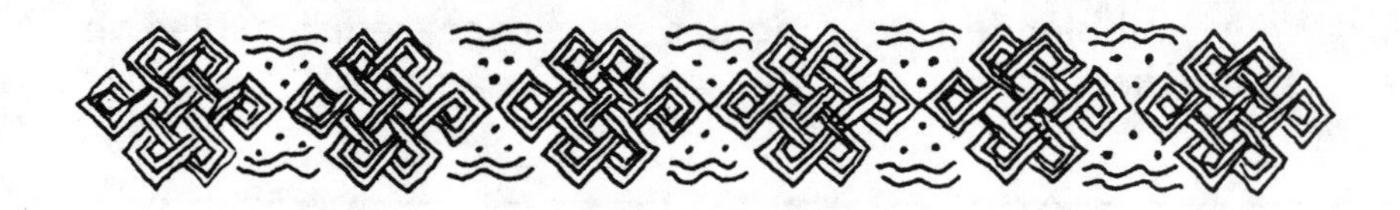

Steamed Bread

- ¾ C. cold water
- 2 T. sugar
- 1 packet dry yeast
- 1 t. baking powder
- 2 C. all-purpose flour
- 6 oz. warm peanut oil

Mix ¾ cup cold water, sugar, and yeast. Add the baking powder and 2 cups of flour, incorporate, and allow to rise for 40 minutes. In another bowl, mix 1 cup flour and ½ cup boiling water. In a third bowl mix 1½ cups flour with warm oil. Knead the flour-yeast mixture, incorporating the flour-and-boiling-water mixture. Knead until smooth (about 5 to 7 minutes) and roll out into a 12-inch x 20-inch rectangle. Using a spatula, spread flour-and-oil mixture over the dough and roll up jelly-roll fashion. Cut into 2-inch sections and place in one layer on a heat-proof plate in a covered steamer. Steam over high heat for 6 to 8 minutes.

6 servings

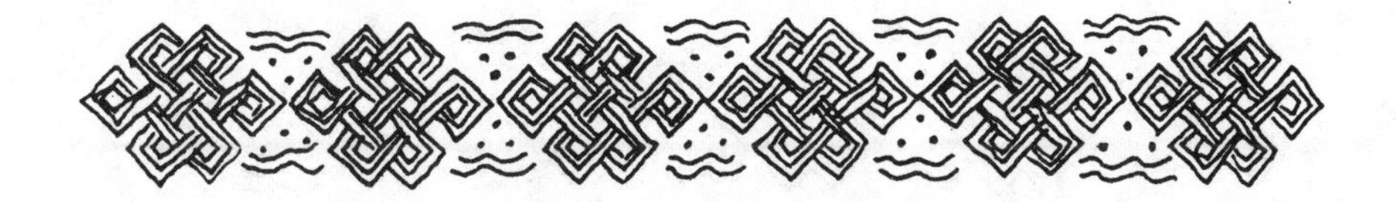

Carp with Hot Bean Sauce

1	whole	carp, approximately 2 lb.
1/2	C.	cooking oil
1	T.	fresh ginger, minced
1	T.	fresh garlic, minced
2	T.	hot bean paste, available in specialty stores
2	T.	soy sauce
2	T.	Shaoxing rice wine (or dry sherry)
1/2	t.	salt
	t.	sugar
1 1/2	C.	water
2	t.	cornstarch dissolved in 1 T. vinegar
1	T.	sesame oil
2	T.	spring onions, chopped

Keep the fish whole and make sure it is well scaled and clean. Cut 3 or 4 diagonal slashes 1/4-inch deep on each side. Heat a *wok*, add 1/4 cup of the oil, and swirl it around the *wok*. Add the fish and fry it on both sides until crisp and set to the side of the *wok*. Add the remaining oil and stir fry the ginger, garlic, hot bean paste, soy sauce, wine, salt, and sugar. Add the water and cook the fish for 10 minutes. Remove the fish to a warm plate. Reduce the liquid in the pan a bit and add the cornstarch-vinegar mixture, sesame oil, and spring onions. Blend, pour over the fish, and serve immediately. *6 servings*

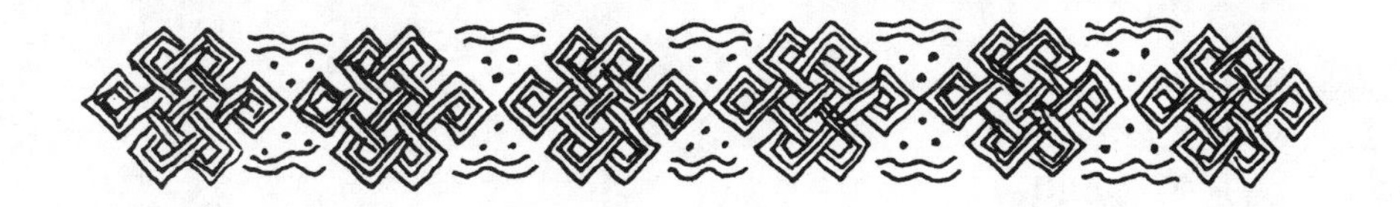

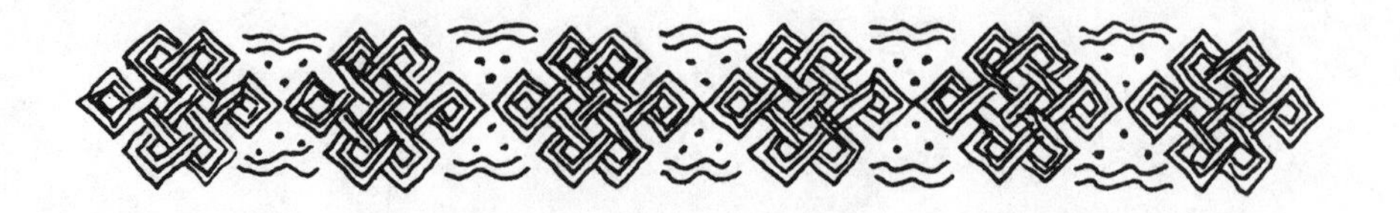

Sweet Potato Croquettes

8	oz.	sweet potatoes
1	oz.	lard
4	oz.	glutinous-rice flour
8	oz.	sweet red-bean paste
2–3	oz.	sesame seeds
		oil for deep frying

Peel and cube the sweet potatoes and steam until tender. Mash the sweet potatoes with lard. Spread on a flat surface and knead in the glutinous-rice flour to make a smooth mixture. Divide the mixture into 24 portions. Spread out the sweet red-bean paste and form into 24 olive-sized portions. Flatten one portion of soft dough on the palm of your hand, place the bean paste in the center, and close the dough around it. Roll in sesame seeds and fry until golden brown. Drain and serve. 6 *servings*

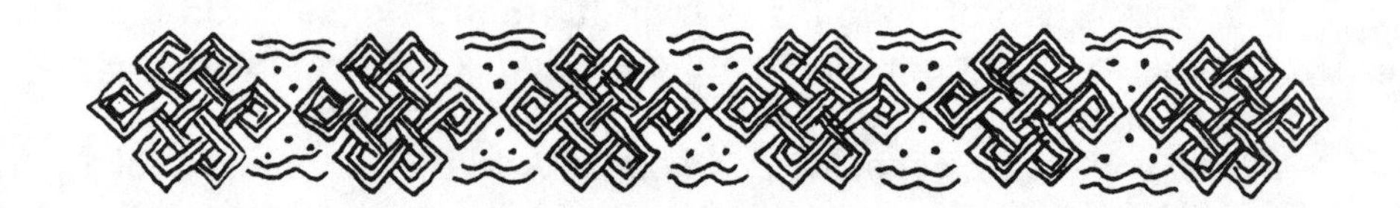

Baked Chinese Tapioca

1½	C.	Chinese tapioca
10	C.	water
1	C.	sugar
2	C.	water
3	T.	butter

1	C.	milk
5	T.	cornstarch dissolved in 6 T. cold water
3		egg yolks
1	t.	vanilla extract
1	C.	red-bean paste
1	T.	butter

Preheat the oven to 425°. Fill a pan with 10 cups of water, bring it to a boil, add the tapioca, lower the heat, and cook for 5 minutes or until the tapioca becomes transparent. Drain the tapioca and reserve. In a pot large enough to hold all the ingredients, boil together 2 cups of water and the sugar for 3 minutes, then add the 3 tablespoons of butter and milk. Thicken the mixture with the cornstarch paste and turn off the heat. Add the vanilla and egg yolks and stir briskly. Add the tapioca and blend well. Roll the sweet red-bean paste into a circle ½-inch thick. Place half of the tapioca mixture in a baking dish. Place the layer of bean paste over it and top with the remainder of the tapioca mixture. Dot with 1 tablespoon of butter. Bake for 15 minutes until the surface becomes golden. *6 servings*

Persimmons

9

HERBAL SPECIALTIES

When Shen Neng (3494 B.C.E.), the legendary emperor, introduced agriculture to the people of China, he bound it, at the same time to both culinary and medicine applications, since he had tested and recorded the benefits and toxins of a multitude of flora and fauna. He is also credited with the idea of opposing principles, still defined as "yin" and "yang." As early as the Shang Dynasty, the bronze cauldron was an important insignia of the imperial household, and one chef was even made prime minister.

By 500 B.C.E. specific plant, animal, and mineral ingredients were recognized as elements of pharmacology. Confucius (551–479 B.C.E.) treated food as an integral part of his outlook. In the East and the West apothecaries and herbalists were one and the same for centuries, and it is only in most recent times that the two have become divided (if not to say divisive in the West). In 450 B.C.E. Hippocrates, the father of modern Western medicine, told of 400 herbs in his pharmacy. Herbs have been used by practitioners of diverse philosophies and religions throughout the world.

Lao Tzu (Laozi "The Old Boy") dealt with a spiritual destination and for centuries it has been debated whether the "tao" or "path" is the journey or the arrival. In the Taoist tradition it is believed that the "Herb of Immortality" grows on the "Island of the Eastern Sea." He, too, acknowledged the yin and yang in the striving for harmony through diet as well as outlook. Though moderation was recommended, the organs of animals were prescribed in tonic form to strengthen the corresponding organ in the person using it.

The physician's job was in large part preventive advice. Bian Qu (407–310 B.C.E.) is considered to be the first doctor, but more is known about Zhang Zhongjing, the author of "Shang Han Lun" (200 B.C.E.), "A Treatise on Fevers." The work includes observation on acupuncture, body meridians, surgery, and narcotic anesthesia as it was practiced then. He describes the use of cinnamon, ginger, jujubes, licorice in one tonic, and lists eighty others. In China, licorice root extract continues to be used as a base for many herbal medicines and often as a sweetener to make some ingredients more palatable. Studies now at Duke University show it to be a detoxifier and some go so far as to say that the triterpenoids it contains will cause pre-cancerous cells to develop normally.

Even people using the most modern medicine heed traditional medicine as well. It was discovered by American researchers that shark cartilage had anti-carcinogen properties. Genuine bird's nest soup is regarded as soothing and nutritious for people with some stomach conditions like ulcers. The nests are made from predigested protein as the alkaline fluids in the birds' mouths break down the elements in the seaweed used by the petrel that lives high on South Pacific cliffs. So while we look askance at some of the ingredients, it is good to bear in mind that some have been tested for hundreds, and in some cases, thousands, of years.

Green tea is said not only to lower cholesterol and blood pressure but block the activity of many carcinogens. More research is being done both in this country and China.

In the West, everything from Omega 3 fatty acids in fish or flaxseed to prevent or even reverse plaque buildup in blood vessels to the sterol in cucumbers, said to assist in the elimination of cholesterol from the body, has been backed by statistical analysis.

China uses almost no dairy products and instead many legume derivatives as "milk" drinks. There are many delicious forms of *dofu* and other soy products. Now soy milk and *dofu* have become popular in this country and are used nationwide. Scientific studies have revealed that eating tofu in large portions will decrease cholesterol.

Cornell University has done a China study on Health and Nutrition that has shown a combination of low-fat high-fiber, herbal medicine and exercise like Tai Chi has produced great benefits. In East and West the combination of modern and traditional practices has become a practical example of yin and yang. The physician's job was, in large part, to give preventive advice.

Zhang Zhongjing, an early Chinese writer on well-being, talks also of "Qi" which means both energy and matter and is regarded as a vital force (*elan vital*). It is not unusual in Chinese for substance and function to be the same word.

In the Han Dynasty (206 B.C.E.–220 C.E.), yin and yang were formalized and balance was sought in most activities. Five became an important number—the senses of sight, sound, taste, touch, and smell. The five elements were defined as water, fire, wood, metal, and earth, and the five blessings as longevity, prosperity, health (physical and mental), virtue, and a death befitting a good life. The five directions, North, East, South, West, and Center, were likened to the five tastes and to parts of the body; sweetness for the spleen, sourness the liver, hotness the lungs, bitterness the heart, saltiness the kidneys.

Of course the seasons, the climate, the cooking fires, and the combinations of food, all affect physical needs and the foods that bring the most benefit.

In the Banpo Neolithic Museum are tortoise shells and animal bones inscribed with recipes for food to feed the sick, as well as prayers for their well-being. It also has tripod cooking vessels dating from 7000 B.C.E. And yet China's history has virtually no general proscriptions or taboos against any food. It is one of the most inclusive cuisines in the world.

Some aspects of yang are heaven (*ch'ien*), male, and also whatever is perceived as strong and increasing like the sun, fire, heat, spring, summer, and beginnings. Yin is, among other things, earth (*k'un*), female, and what is perceived as harmonious, tranquil, nourishing, and sustaining like the moon, cold, water, fall, winter, and completion. Together they affect growth and change in the world because they produce and reproduce. So many dishes today include at least the yin of spring onion and the yang of ginger.

The comingling of scientific and gastronomic curiosity is not so odd a concept. It has led to an exquisite cuisine that always acknowledges the nutritional potential in all food.

Sometimes the benefit seems a metaphor. The perseverance of a carp, the strength of a tiger, the tranquility of dragon's bone, amber and vegetables. "What pleases the palate will please the mind" is an old Chinese adage. Sometimes it seems to me that the reverse is also true and that what pleases the mind will please the palate.

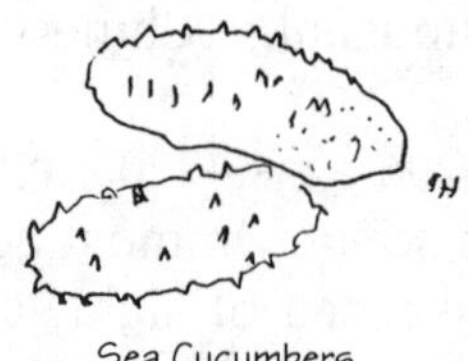

Sea Cucumbers

The smooth gelatinous jellyfish and the sea slug, usually called *bêche-de-mer* in French, or sea cucumber in English, are regarded as good moisturizers for the skin and are considered anti-aging.

By the T'ang Dynasty (618–907 C.E.) there were medical colleges, and tonics and soups made from snake were part of medicinal and culinary writing. Some Westerners are surprised to learn that not only in many Native American groups was snake eaten, but that in the southwestern area of the United States it is still served in some gourmet restaurants. In the last century extracts used to be made into "Snake Oil Elixir" and peddled from town to town. Maybe they were better than we give them credit for.

In China, wine made from snake bile is considered a good winter drink to alleviate aches, pains, and impotence. Venom is extracted to make serum of various kinds. Snake gall bladder is used to relieve symptoms of rheumatism.

The following recipe is courtesy of the Hong Kong Tourist Association.

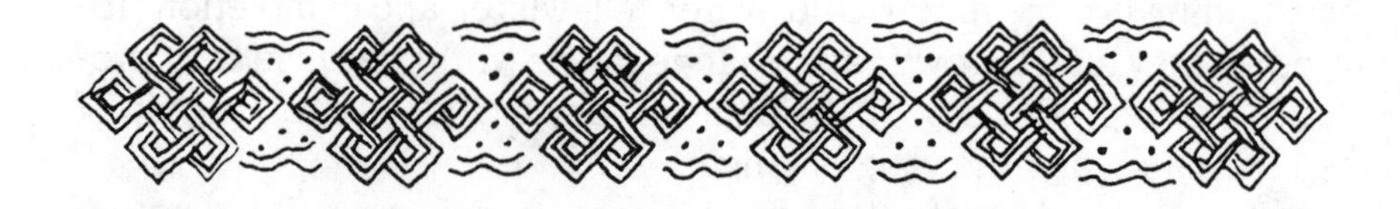

Shredded Chicken and Snake Soup

12 oz.	frozen snake fillet
1	chicken, 2½ to 3 lb.
1½	inch piece of fresh ginger, peeled
8	dried black mushrooms (soaked)

2		strips tangerine peel
1	oz.	dried black fungus (soaked and cooked)
2	oz.	ginger, peeled and shredded
8	oz.	fish maw
2	T.	sesame oil
1		inch piece ginger, peeled
4		spring onions, minced
2	T.	Shaoxing wine
1		inch piece of ginger peeled
10	C.	chicken and snake broth

Seasoning

2	T.	light soy sauce
1	T.	dark soy sauce
2	t.	sugar
1	t.	white pepper
		salt to taste

Thickening

8	T.	water chestnut powder
3/4	C.	water

Garnish

4		fresh lemon leaves (1 t. grated lemon zest may be substituted)
1	oz.	parsley

Defrost the snake fillet and plunge into 3 cups of boiling water for 10 minutes with 1 1/2 inch piece of ginger. Drain. Then cook in 8–10 cups of water for 1 1/2 hours. Drain and retain 4–5 cups of water for later use. Shred the fillet finely. Boil the chicken in 10 cups of water with the other piece of ginger. Cook for 2 1/2 hours. Reserve broth. Debone and shred the chicken.

Cut mushrooms, tangerine peel, and black fungus into slivers. Cook shredded ginger in 1 cup of boiling water, drain and run under cold water.

Heat the sesame oil in a small, heavy saucepan. Add another 1 inch piece of ginger, minced spring onions, Shaoxing wine, and 2 cups of water. Add the fish maw and cook for 15 minutes. Shred the fish maw.

Discard liquid.

Put the snake and chicken broth together, totaling 10 cups, in a stockpot and heat. Add all the shredded ingredients and the seasoning and simmer. In a small bowl, stir the water chestnut powder into 3/4 cup water until dissolved and then stir into the soup. Add parsley and lemon leaves or lemon zest. Do not boil. Serve as hot as possible. *8 servings*

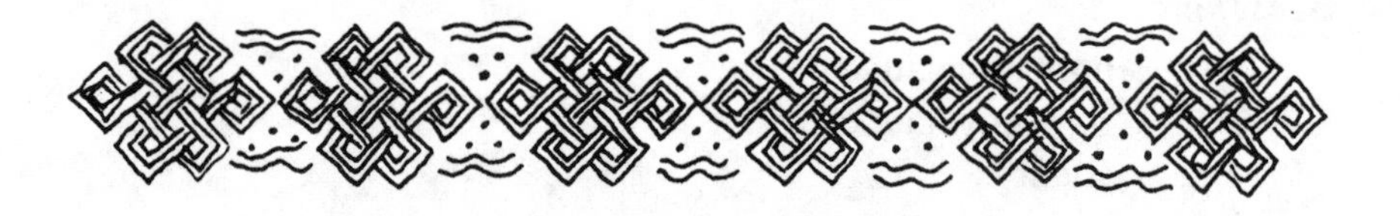

In Taipei I met with Clark Hsieh, a professor and chairman of the School of Nutrition & Health Science at the Taipei Medical College and the president of the Chinese Nutrition Society, and Kuo-Tung-Chen, a professor in the School of Pharmacy, Taipei Medical College. We talk, in English and Chinese, with a translator.

They emphasize that the Departments of Nutrition and Pharmacy are part of the medical team that manages both hospital and outpatient care. In addition to addressing the usual array of ailments that are presented to hospital staffs every day, they research the topics of stress, hypertension, obesity, and general issues of illness and wellness, in both traditional and modern Eastern and Western medicine. We discuss fast food and the chemistry of garlic and ginger.

One of their suggestions is to eat meals with dishes arranged from light to heavy, then finish with more light ones. Many people say that after they eat Chinese food they are soon hungry again. It seems to me that this is a benefit. A good meal is not supposed to make you feel as though you swallowed a basketball. Often, cultures eat worse as they become modernized. Overprocessing has lowered the nutritive value of many dishes. As white flour and sugar, instant rice and noodle dishes enter the marketplace, meals high in sodium and fat, low in fruit, vegetables, and fiber content dominate. Fast food franchises aren't helping as hamburgers, fries, and sweet desserts now offer understandable ease and instant gratification.

There has been a lot of negative talk about the use of fat in Chinese cooking, but it is used and eaten in such small amounts and in combination with so much that is nutritionally sound that the good has far outweighed the bad. The MSG that is being phased out has only been used for about twenty years, and though it causes headaches to some, has shown no lasting side effects. The Out Patient Department trend is toward fewer prescription drugs and more nutrition and lifestyle changes, especially for hypertension which is on the rise for the first time in Asia. The whole team plans a regime and follows up on each patient. Though they offer vitamin and mineral supplements, the rampant excessive use of them without knowledge or supervision might be risky.

The Chief of Pharmacology comes in and speaks to me in English and to the rest of the group in Chinese. When he starts using the blackboard to explain chemical reactions, I am fascinated, but explain that I have had only a year of chemistry in high school. We laugh, but he continues. For ten minutes I can actually follow it.

According to tradition, garlic is a warming and pungent food that is a tonic for energy, respiration, and digestion. It also "aerates" the body, a quality which is described as preventing dampness from settling in to cause colds and offer hospitality to various bugs and parasites. Customarily garlic is recommended to be eaten regularly, but in moderation, because an excess is considered harmful for the stomach and liver.

We talk about the difference between fresh garlic and garlic extracts and supplements. He explains that it is not merely the contents of the garlic, but the chemical interaction it has within the body that gives its greatest benefit. There has been much research on the chemistry of garlic that indicates it inhibits thromboses. It contains allicin, allithiamin, and anasulfides. During cooking garlic produces alinamine, thiamine, and propyldisulfate.

Many of the herbs work in slow ways, as trace active ingredients act as progressive restoratives. With very small long-term doses, effects such as strengthening immunities or relieving ailments can be seen. Under professional supervision it has been shown to be a viable alternative to regulating symptoms in some illnesses. There is a very low incidence of allergic reactions to it.

Ginseng has been used for ages in China. What is interesting is that now the most sought after variety is imported to China from Wisconsin. Ginseng roots are generally cultivated for several years and then cleaned and preserved in various ways. Primarily used as a longevity tonic, it is made up into tea, soup, capsules, and dried slivers that can be used in cooking. It is used to increase energy and therefore should be used with caution by people with elevated blood pressure or any cardiovascular symptoms. It also has plant estrogen and may excite the hormones in ways that aren't beneficial. That said, under supervision it has been used to aid in digestion and is an antidiuretic. I know it is highly touted, but it is something that I think should not be taken without professional inquiries.

In Shanghai, at the Sheraton Hua Ting, Tsang Han Fai, one of the best and most knowledgeable chefs I have ever encountered, presides at the rooftop restaurant Guan Yue Tai (Palace for Appreciating the Moon) . The restaurant has been featuring an extraordinary specialty that he has designed. The menu is a modern version of a traditional Chinese meal featuring medicinal herbs and ingredients. It is a ten- or twelve-course meal, individually plated, and using for each dish, ingredients served both for their taste and enhancement of well-being. The music is supplied by the quartet of Zeng, Pipa, Erh Hu, and Yang Qing which sounds very pleasing and a little like a Philip Glass suite.

This herbal dinner is based on ancient Chinese cuisine, with the intention that the sundry ingredients selected will balance yin and yang and harmonize organs and their functions. It also assures a fine appearance to the skin and increased vim and vigor.

We start with the traditional cold plate, designated on the menu as the Assorted Herbal Platter. It contains: shredded chicken breast, fine black moss, cucumber (to moisturize the lungs), black mushroom, ginger (yang, a digestion aid and good for blood circulation), wolfberry (*gouqizi*—nourishes yin, lowers blood pressure, and improves eyesight), glossy ganoderma (*ling chih*—also known as the immortality fungus which offers longevity and wisdom) and the lilyturf root (*maimendong*—nourishes yin and strengthens the stomach). It is said that eating this assortment with some frequency promotes a healthy body and a long life.

A surprisingly tasty dish is a combination of Mountain Ginseng, Sea Cucumber, and Caterpillar Fungus which is prepared with sea cucumber which nourishes the spirit and is anti-aging, bamboo shoot that has a cold energy to balance the heat of meat, and Jin Hua ham which is said to help heal wounds. This dish is stewed with fresh white mushrooms and is reputed to build up energy, relieve coughs, and reduce phlegm.

We have Deep Fried Quail. Quail nourishes and strengthens the function of the heart, liver, spleen, lungs, and kidneys. It is seasoned with an abundance of fried garlic which lowers blood pressure and kills viruses.

Some of the other dishes can be prepared in the home kitchen since most of the ingredients are available at Chinese specialty food stores which are carrying an ever increasing array of distinctive products.

The following recipes are presented in an unconventional form so that the reader has some idea of the function of many specialized ingredients and some idea of how to deal with them.

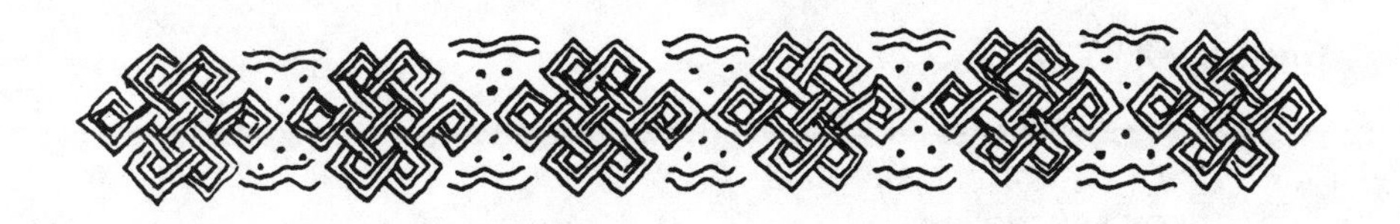

Cold Dish of Chicken, Jellyfish, and Mushroom

1½ C. **diagonally sliced celery (said to lower blood pressure)**

3 **medium carrots (good for eyes, skin, hair) Scrape, score lengthwise with a channel knife, or make V grooves with a paring knife. Slice. Bring water to a boil, add carrot slices and boil for 10 minutes, then drain and set aside.**

1/2 C.	golden needle (dried daylily buds—nourishes lungs, strengthens body) Soak in tepid water for 20 minutes. Drain, discard tips, shred, and reserve.
12	dried black mushrooms (counters carcinogens) Snip off stems and reserve for another use. Pour boiling water over mushroom caps and soak for 30 minutes. Carefully remove from water, making sure any grit has sunk to the bottom. Slice and taste. If there is any grit, rinse them clean, drain, and reserve.
8	ounces of jellyfish (treats colds) Jellyfish is packaged, whole it looks like a golden brown disc, shredded, like a pickled vegetable. If you buy it whole, the easiest way to shred it is to roll it up and sliver it into strips less than 1/4" wide. It will expand in liquid.

Bring a small pot of water to a boil and add jellyfish. Simmer for three or four minutes, drain, and rinse for three or four minutes. Set in a large bowl of cold water, cover, and soak for 6 hours or overnight. When ready to serve, drain and blot with paper towels to dry.

1	whole roasted chicken (strengthens the body)

Garnish

	several sprigs of cilantro (fresh coriander)
4	spring onions, slivered
	soy sauce cruet
	vinegar cruet

When ready to serve, slice chicken and arrange all ingredients artfully on a serving platter. Accompany it with garnish.
Function: reduces high blood pressure and fights obesity.

6 servings

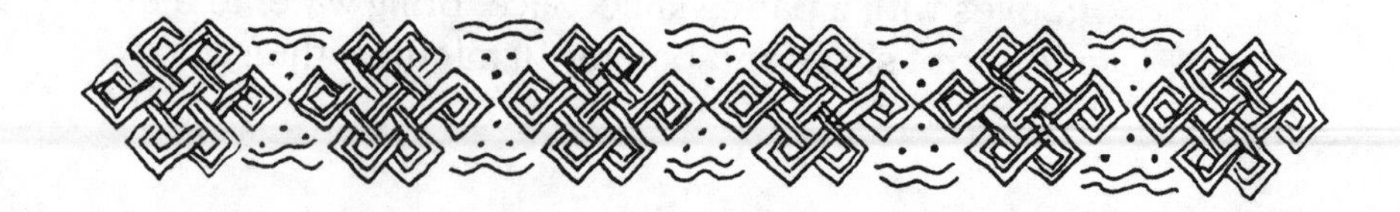

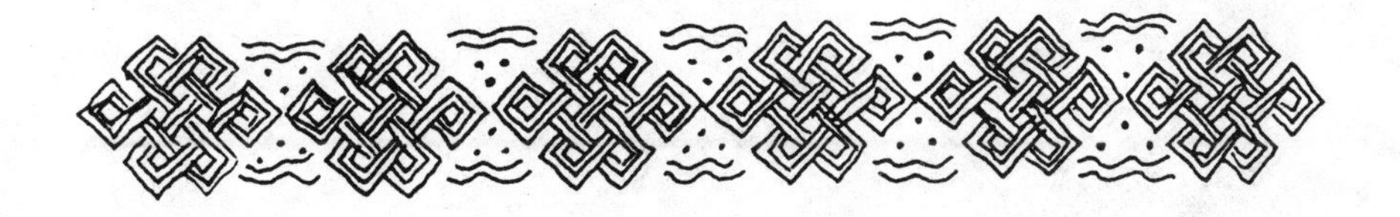

Boiled Beef in Spicy Sauce and Chinese Herbs

1½	lb.	beef brisket or bottom round
3	oz.	*deng shen* root (*codonopsis tangshen*, counters fatigue)
2	oz.	*huang qi* root (*astragalus membranaceus*, lowers blood pressure)
2	oz.	*gancao* (licorice root, counteracts toxins and fatigue)
½	oz.	star anise (relieves abdominal discomfort and cold symptoms)
1	oz.	*rougui* (cassia/cinnamon, aids digestion, calms nerves)
1	oz.	*cao guo* (amomum seed, prevents stomach distension)
1	oz.	bay leaf
½	oz.	*dingxiang* (clove, aids digestion)
1	oz.	dried orange peel (remedy for gas, belching, water retention)
¼	t.	salt
1	t.	sugar

Trim brisket. Mix all other ingredients together and rub meat as best you can. Place all ingredients that do not adhere to the brisket in 2 quarts of water in *wok* or dutch oven and bring to a boil. Place brisket in boiling water and simmer 1½ hours or until tender. Remove brisket from pot and drain. Slice and place on serving dish.

Function: builds up Qi and is good for kidneys. *6 servings*

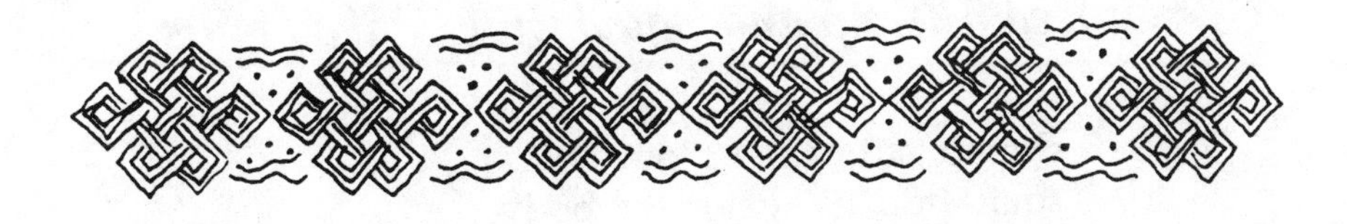

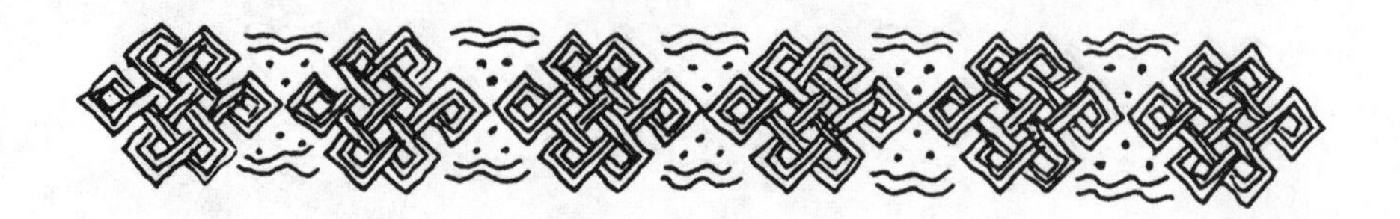

Sauteed Chicken with Pine Nuts

8 oz. boneless chicken breast
2 T. cooking oil
2 oz. pine nuts (lubricates throat and lungs, moistens skin)
1 t. fresh ginger, minced
2 small dried whole chili peppers
1/4 C. chicken broth
2 spring onions, minced
2 t. sesame oil

Cut chicken along the grain into 1 1/2-inch pieces. Heat cooking oil in *wok* or skillet and add chicken and pine nuts, stir for 30 seconds, and add ginger and chili peppers and stir for 30 seconds. Pour broth over all and stir till well blended. Cook for 1 minute and add spring onions and sesame oil. Stir and cook for 2 minutes and serve.

Function: nourishes yin, relieves heat in body, stimulates appetite, invigorates the function of the spleen. *2 servings*

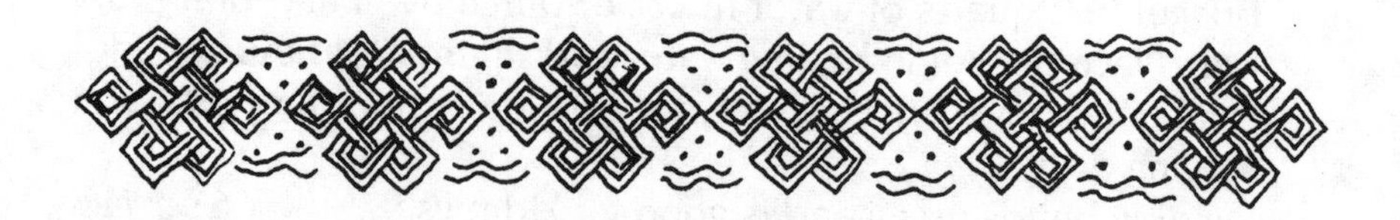

Sauteed Shrimp and Squid with Ginkgo Nuts

1/2 lb. shrimp (strengthens lower back)
1/2 lb. squid (retains heat in the body)
2 oz. ginkgo nuts (*baiguo*, settles Qi, fights thirst)
1 carrot, diced

1 T. minced ginger
1 T. garlic, minced
1 oz. salad oil
salt
sugar
1 t. cornstarch mixed in 2 T. water

Bring 2 quarts of water to a boil and add the shrimp, squid, and ginkgo nuts. Boil for 5 minutes and drain under cold water. Heat the oil in a *wok* or skillet and stir the ginger and garlic until fragrant.
Function: smooths Qi and stimulates appetite. *4 servings*

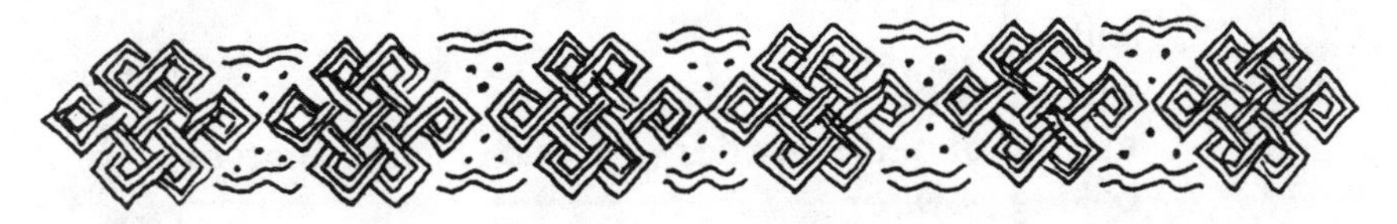

Double-Boiled Black Chicken with Ginseng

½ black bone chicken (a regular chicken may be substituted)
2 oz. Jin Hua ham
2 oz. pork, diced
3 T. ginseng, shredded
1 T. ginger, minced
salt

Using a cleaver for chopping, cut the chicken into small pieces, leaving the bone and skin on. Blanch the chicken, ham, and pork in boiling water for a minute or two. Drain them and put them in a 3-quart heat proof bowl with ginseng, ginger, and salt and 6 cups of water. Place bowl uncovered on steamer rack, cover steamer, and steam for 2 hours.
Function: builds Qi, relieves heat, and helps produce saliva.
2 *servings*

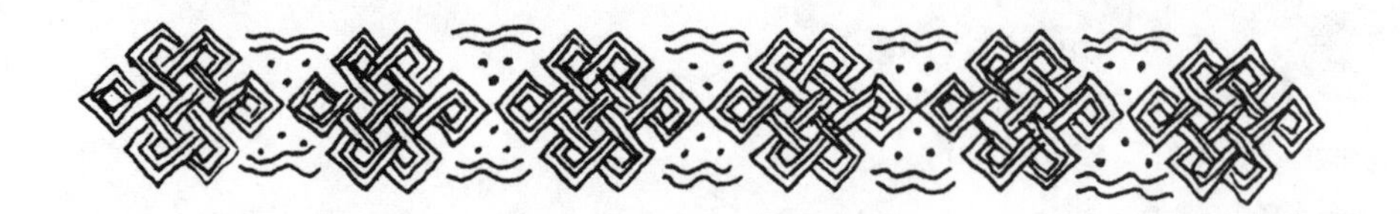

Deep-Fried Scallops

1	lb.	scallops
1		egg
2	T.	water
½	C.	all purpose flour
½	t.	salt
¼	t.	white pepper
1	T.	mother of pearl powder (*zhenzhumu*, calms nerves)
2	t.	baking powder
4	C.	oil for deep frying or according to manufacturer's directions for electric fryer
1		cucumber (peeled, cut in half lengthwise, seeded, and cut into slices)

Rinse scallops and trim to uniform size, if necessary. Mix together egg and water. Mix together flour, salt and pepper, mother of pearl powder, and baking powder.

Heat oil in fryer.

Dip scallops in egg mixture. Dip in dry mixture. Fry in hot oil for 3 minutes and serve immediately with cucumber slices.

Function: benefits liver, calms nerves, and relieves fever and insomnia.

4 servings

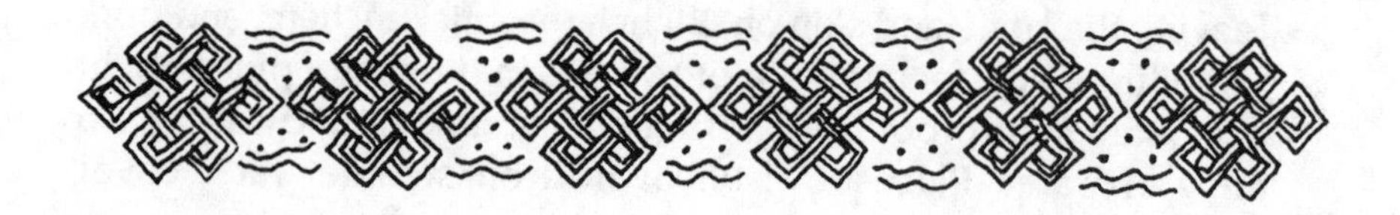

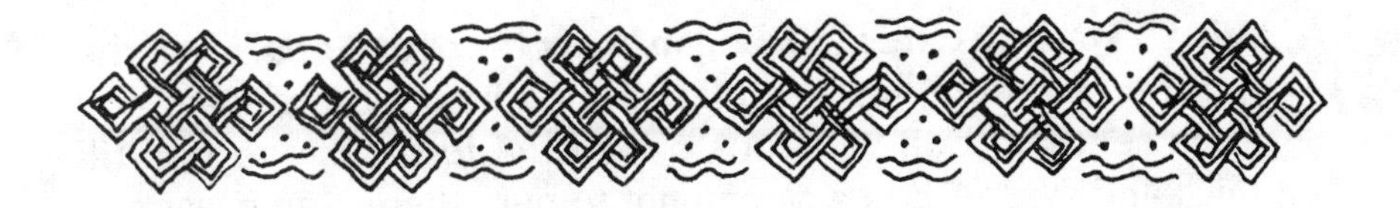

Fried Rice with Garlic and Assorted Meat

3 T.	cooking oil
6	cloves of garlic, minced
1/4 lb.	boneless cooked skinless chicken breast, diced
1/4 lb.	shelled medium cooked shrimp, diced
1	egg (cooked into an omelet and cut into strips)
1	carrot, scraped and diced
4	spring onions, diced
1 lb.	steamed rice
	salt

Heat cooking oil in *wok* and stir garlic until it starts to brown. Add ingredients one by one to hot oil and stir till well browned and blended. When all ingredients are incorporated be certain everything in the *wok* is hot. Serve immediately.

Function: cleanses the system. *6 servings*

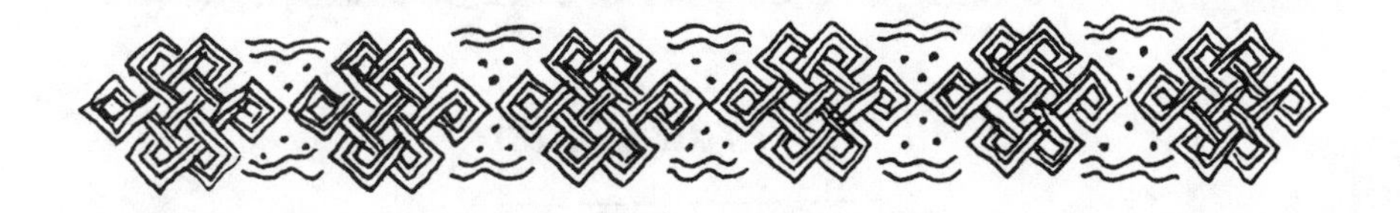

Double-Boiled Three Kinds of Dates with Crystal Sugar

1/2 C.	red dates (energy tonic)
1/2 C.	dark dates (benefits the blood)
1/2 C.	jujube, (nourishes the blood, soothes the mind)
1/4 C.	lotus seeds (calmative)
1/2 C.	crystal sugar

Bring 3 kinds of dates to a boil in water to cover. Put a lid on the pot, remove from heat, and let sit for 2 hours. Bring sugar and lotus seeds to boil in 2 cups of water. Add dates and boil till thick and syrupy, being careful not to burn them. Serve warm or cold.

6 servings

Function: enriches blood, preserves appearance, and benefits lungs

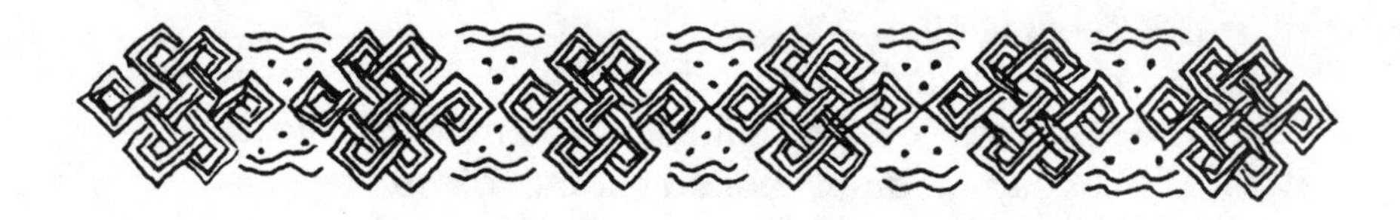

Tea

American ginseng, prepared according to proportions given on package.

Function: builds up Qi, preserves yin, relieves heat.

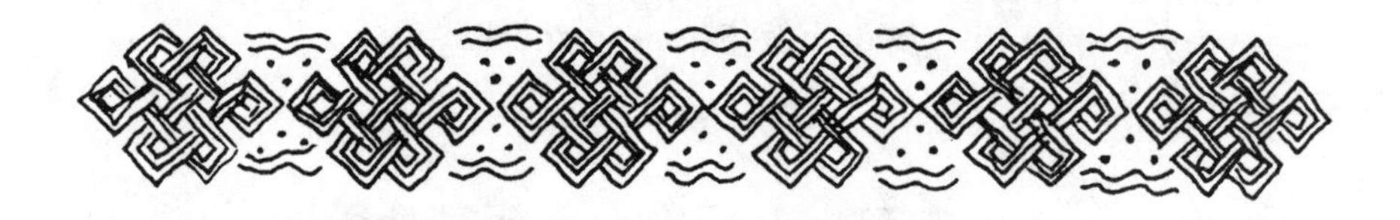

Fresh Fruit Platter

watermelon (promotes urination)
hami melon (detoxicates the blood)
grapes (energy tonic, benefits bones and muscles)
mandarin apple
pear (prevents indigestion)
star fruit (anti cough and fever of cold, detoxicates)
kiwi fruit (high in vitamin C)

Select the above fruit in any combination, when ripe. Wash fruit and slice it into decorative pieces. Arrange on platter.

10

Vegetarian Cuisine

From simple cabbage dishes to elaborate banquets where vegetables become the centers of attention, vegetables are, after grain, the dominant food of China. Whether they are prepared in country households where a pot or two fills all culinary needs or in grand restaurants where they are served in the elegant court style, the selection, preparation, cooking, and serving of vegetables is always treated respectfully in China. They are never served with excuses, because it would never occur to anyone that they are secondary to any other ingredient, except perhaps rice.

For 2,500 years, not only vegetables but vegetarianism has been touted by many. Some extol them without a philosophical view, simply finding it expedient and "natural" to eat vegetables. Eventually Buddhist and Taoist teaching proscribed vegetables in various specific forms and degrees. To this day, some of the best vegetarian meals are cooked in temple kitchens by monks or nuns who combine tradition with modern means.

The soybean, which contains twice the protein of meat, has been a vegetable staple for ages. Not only the ubiquitous sprout, but the bean is processed into myriad forms of *dofu* (bean curd). It has a versatility that has put it on shopping lists all over the world. In China *dofu* is prepared and served in many ways: soft and custardy, springy and chewy, dried and seasoned like meat or chicken, spiced and fried, and sweet or savory. The *fu chu* (bean curd skin) can be used for everything from spring roll wrappers to crisp duck skin.

Mushrooms are another large presence in vegetable cuisine. Fresh, dried, or preserved, they range from tiny baby mushrooms to the large black mushrooms, that are frequently dried. Fungi are cultivated forms of mushrooms that have names that translate to "cloud ear," "wood ear," and more because of the shapes they have as they grow. Sea-moss fungus is often mistaken for slivers of seaweed but *fa*

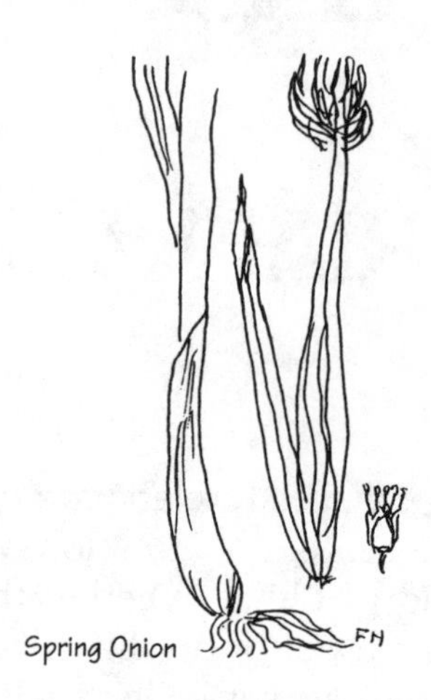

Spring Onion

tsai is related to the other fungi and is favored in New Year's dishes. One reason is that its name resembles *fat choy*, which means "to grow in riches."

Nutrition and health have played an important part in the general preparation of vegetables in China. It is still rare to see them served raw. Instead they are usually well cleaned, trimmed, and quickly steamed or stir fried to retain their vitamins and minerals. Often they are cooked with ginger and/or garlic, which have many healthful properties. Now, with the benefit of refrigeration, some are cooled and served as cold dishes. They are specially good this way with the addition of some Chinkiang vinegar and/or a splash of sesame oil. Recipes for slow-cooked, braised vegetable stews and soups date back ages. In the Han Dynasty bamboo shoots, leeks, and turnip stews were recorded.

By the T'ang Dynasty, bamboo was so appreciated as a food that large sections of gardens and cookbooks were devoted to it. Winter shoots are the smallest, followed in size by the spring shoots. The bamboo shoots of summer are the ones, no doubt, that Marco Polo praised as having the shape and texture of asparagus. It is the central portion of the shoot that is edible, and it must be prepared with care, parboiled to eliminate the bitter and toxic hydrocyanic acid. It is often sold in markets ready to eat. Once it has been stripped of any leaves, its outer rind, and base, it should be boiled for about twenty minutes before adding to other dishes. It can then be refrigerated or frozen until needed.

Nasturtium, now so popular in the West, was equally popular in China until it fell out of use. Contemporary chefs are bringing it back into favor.

Carved and shaped vegetables continue to decorate the plates of banquet and restaurant plates, as well as special home-cooked dishes. Carrots, melons, tomatoes, radishes, and turnips are carved, and other vegetables are sliced and shaped to form fantasies of flora and fauna. Many vegetables are dried, pickled, and preserved in a variety of ways and are incorporated into many dishes as well as eaten as accompaniments.

One place to enjoy a monastery meal is in Hong Kong. The ferry from Central in Hong Kong to Lantau Island's Po Lin Temple takes an hour, and the bus ride is another 45 minutes from Silvermine Bay. There, the famous large, outdoor bronze Buddha invites reflection as lunch is eaten in the refectory.

In Taiwan with a guide and translator, I drive to Kuanyin Mountain and The Temples Between the Clouds. It is a place I am introducing to them; although I have never been there I have read about it. There is an unbelievable vista—on the one side is a panoramic view of T'aipei and on the other is the top of the mountain, looking like the craggy peaks we have seen in Chinese landscape paintings, and the beautiful temple.

First we must eat, because food is served only from noon to 1:00, when it is cleared away. In a low-ceilinged cement-finished room the size of a large hotel lobby there is, at the doorway, a small shrine of Kuanyin with offerings. In the front of the shrine is a donation box; one gives according to choice. There are thirty round tables surrounded by small, low stools, some wood, some formica and chrome. It is clearly catch-as-catch-can, since only four tables are occupied,

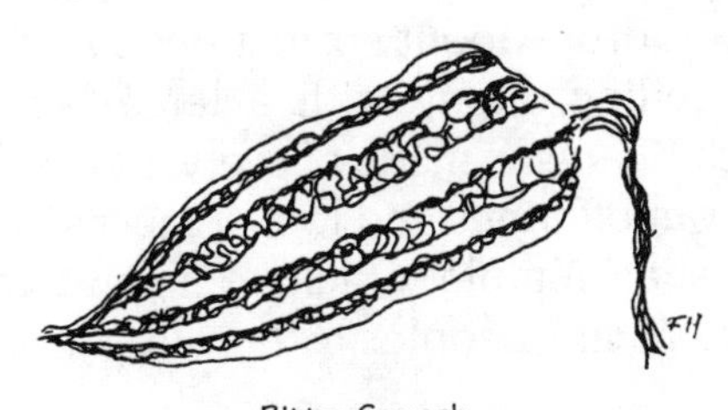

Bitter Squash

mainly by workers doing ongoing repairs, renovations, and additions. You can see the small, large-windowed kitchen, and on two trestle tables are bowls of food and pots of soup, rice, and noodles. There is also a carton of styrofoam bowls and plates and one of individually wrapped chopsticks. We help ourselves. My translator and her colleague, who drove us here, are enjoying this as well. They appreciate its seriousness and its respectful sense of presence and community.

The food is cooked by nuns; a beautiful woman in a traditional gray monk's robe and shaved head has done the entire meal. This sort of Buddhist vegetarian food includes no onions, garlic, or related vegetables. Ginger and roots flavor our soup which features great mushrooms and *Dong Kui*—a strength giving herb blend. We eat a dish made of dried mushrooms and glutinous rice and another of sweet potato leaves lightly braised in ginger with a bit of red pepper. There are also carrots sliced with *cai luo bo*, a vegetable root that is described to me as a little like the root of a tree; it stays crunchy even though well-cooked. *Hai cai* (seaweed) is made into a delicious pickle with reduced soy sauce, sugar, and a bit of ginger and red pepper.

We eat surprisingly unselfconsciously, sharing a respect for the food and the environment of its preparation—an acceptance of our presence and of anyone anywhere who joins the meal and makes whatever offering possible to Kuanyin. It is quiet, but by no means hushed. In fact, we talk to the woman who has prepared the food. She picks up morsels with tongs and explains them to me.

At the main altar in the large temple is an enormous statue of Kuanyin with 1,000 arms. I walk around, light incense, meditate, and experience the sober beauty of this place and the people that attend it. The buildings are elaborate structures, simply built of wood and cement, then painted and carved. No pictures are allowed to be taken inside. There appears to be Tibetan writing on the beams of the ceiling, which is divided into squares, each painted with divas and Bodhisattvas among the clouds. There is a *bas-relief* on the back wall of figures in the sky. A drum about six feet deep and fifteen feet across hangs from the ceiling, along with a large bell. There are many smaller altars with Kuanyins made of every material, including porcelain. Fruit and flower offerings and lots of incense fill the temple.

I go to the Lushan Temple, which, to a newcomer, is like a scene from a movie. There are people in the outer courtyard, gift stalls, monks and nuns chanting, and people praying, lighting incense, and burning hell money. The temple has two central enormous altars, around which many other altars are located. There are lots of fruit and food offerings, everything from orchids to Ovaltine. Men, women, and children, who, even to my eye, are from diverse areas, educational backgrounds, and interests, pray and prostrate themselves but mostly everyone is in motion. It is very crowded. Everywhere people are saying beads, chanting, and circumnavigating the shrines repeatedly, as a walking rosary. It is said "The gods do not notice random motion."

For dinner I meet colleagues at the vegeterian Chyun Sheeng Restaurant, and we are seated in a booth that is really a little alcove. It has an open-work shutter on each side that frames the rest of the restaurant. The table is set with celadon-colored cloths and at each place setting are large cloth napkins and a stand on which rest chopsticks and a round-bowled spoon.

We talk about changes in vegetarian cuisine, including its language. No one wants "vegetarian duck" anymore; the mere mention of an animal has become distasteful to purists, and no longer does the comparison reflect the chef's skill at emulating an expected taste and texture. Dishes are being renamed.

We start the meal with various small cold plates. One dish appears to be slices of dried sausage, but are rolls of dried *dofu* skins, soaked for half an hour and then spread with soy sauce, sugar, vinegar, and a little pepper. The skins are then rolled jellyroll fashion, layering the sheets as with *filo* pastry, sheet after sheet to a thickness of an inch and a half. It is then tied like sausage, dried, and sliced thinly at an angle. The tea we are drinking with our meal is made from roasted sweet potatoes. Next we have a thick soup with mushrooms, *dofu* rolls with black mushroom, and spicy gluten, shaped like a hamburger, sauced, and served with broccoli and sliced corn on the cob. Then comes a cereal cube—rice flour is ground with almonds and peanuts and steamed in carrot sauce. This particular Buddhist vegetarian style does not permit any ingredients from the onion family, so there are no leeks, garlic, or green onions to enhance the sauces. We also have a dish that looks like squid, cross hatched in the traditional way. It is made from rice flour cooked with agar-agar, and the texture fools the palate. It is served with bright green pea sprouts. Dessert is

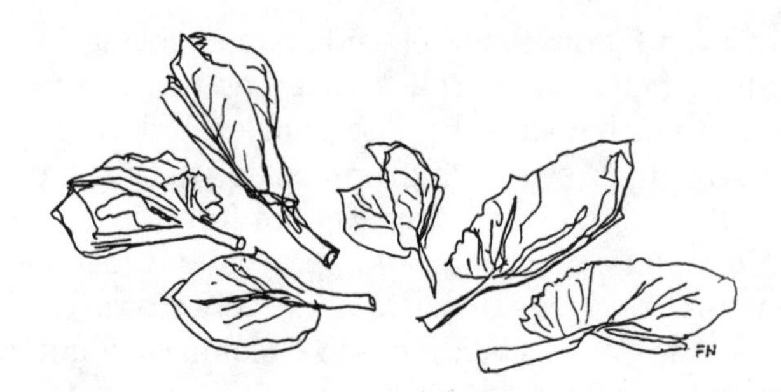

Pea Shoots

a pretty bowl of violet-colored rice powder balls stuffed with sesame paste and served in a sweet sauce.

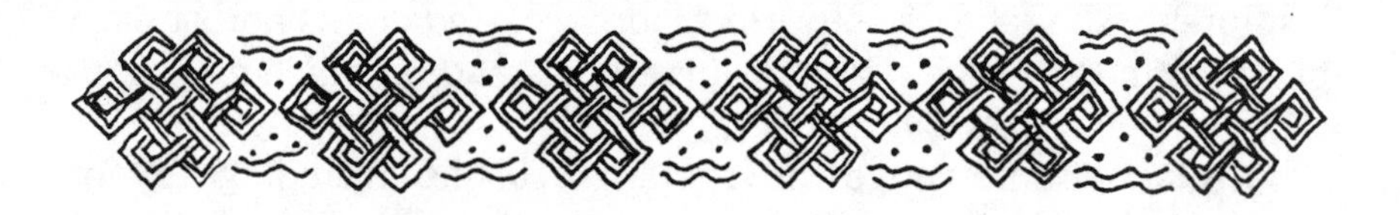

Pea Shoots (Dau Miu)

4 C.	pea shoots (Note: These are delicate tendrils that have a short season and shelf life. They are best used within a day or two of purchase. They have a short stem with two 1-inch oval leaves.)
1 T.	peanut or safflower oil
2 t.	fresh ginger, minced
3	cloves of garlic, minced

Rinse the pea shoots and drain over a paper towel in a colander. Heat the oil in a *wok* or skillet over medium heat. Stir in the ginger and garlic, stir fry in oil until aromatic. Add the pea shoots and stir fry for 2 to 3 minutes. Serve immediately. 2 *servings*

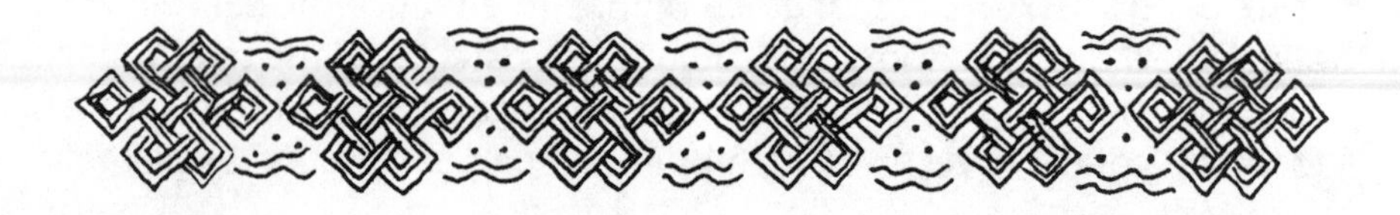

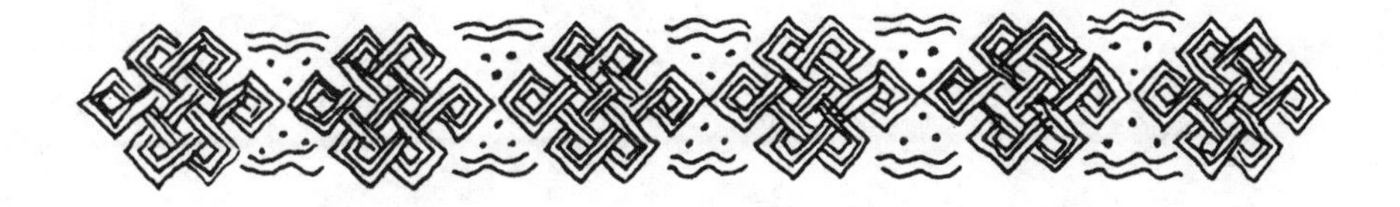

Sichuan Braised Eggplant (Yu Hsiang Ch'ien Zu)

6		narrow Chinese eggplants
1/3	C.	cooking oil
2	t.	fresh ginger, minced
1	T.	fresh garlic, minced
1	T.	chili paste with garlic
2		cakes dry pressed bean curd, diced
4		spring onions, chopped
1	T.	vinegar
2	t.	sesame oil

Wash the eggplants and, without peeling them, remove the stem end and tip. Cut in quarters lengthwise and then into 1-inch pieces. Heat the oil in a *wok* and add the eggplant. Stir and cook for 4 minutes. Remove the eggplant with slotted spoon so that the oil remains in the *wok*. Reserve the eggplant and add the ginger, garlic, chili paste, and bean curd to the *wok*. Stir until well blended, fragrant, and browned. Return the eggplant to the *wok* and stir until the eggplant is limp and the *wok* is almost dry. Add the spring onions, vinegar, and sesame oil and mix for 1 minute. Serve immediately. *2 servings*

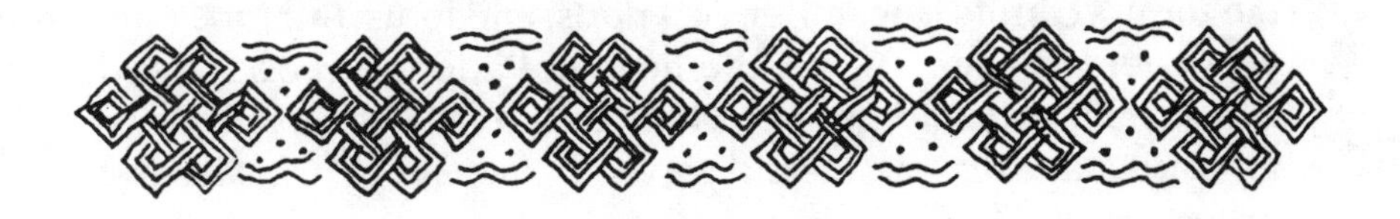

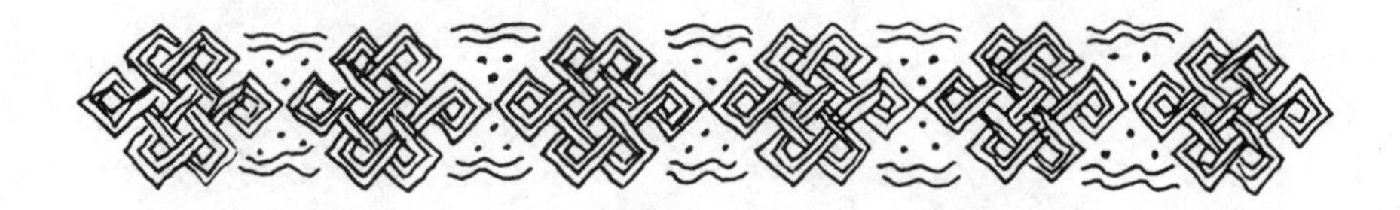

Sauteed Mixed Vegetables (Shih Chin So Hui)

1		medium turnip
2		medium carrots
1		medium cucumber
20		snow pea pods
4	T.	cooking oil
10		fresh black mushrooms, sliced
10		dried black mushrooms, soaked, rinsed, and sliced
8		slices lotus root, blanched in boiling water for 2 minutes
1		*tianjin* cabbage or *bok choi*
20		ginkgo nuts, blanched and peeled
1	t.	brown sugar
		pinch of salt and white pepper to taste
2	t.	cornstarch dissolved in 2 T. cold water
1	T.	oyster sauce
2	t.	sesame oil

Scrape the turnip and carrots and slice decoratively. Do not peel the cucumber; cut it in half lengthwise, remove the seeds, and slice. Trim the snow pea pods. Boil the turnip, carrots, cucumber, and pea pods until tender and crisp, then drain and set aside. Heat the oil in a *wok*, add the mushrooms, and stir. Add the turnip, carrots, cucumber, pea pods, and lotus. Stir for 2 minutes over high heat. Lower the heat and add the cabbage and ginkgo nuts, salt, and pepper. Stir in the cornstarch mixture, oyster sauce, and sesame oil and serve. *4 servings*

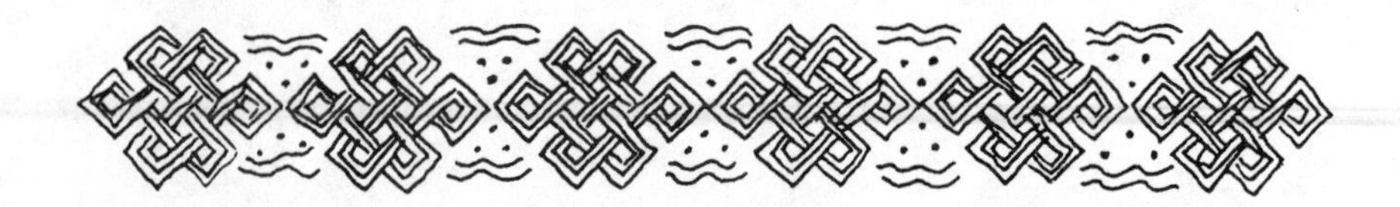

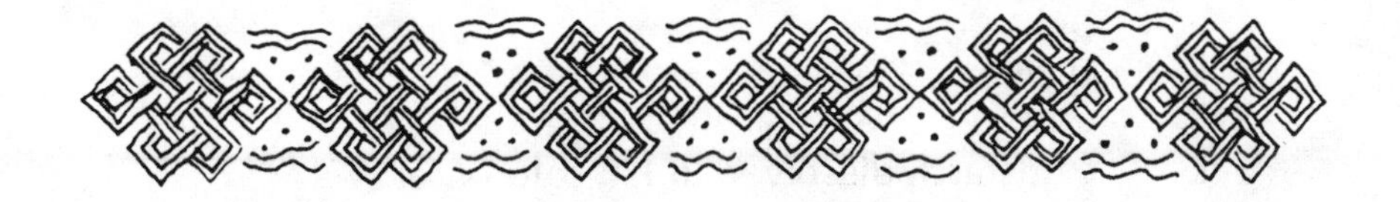

Spicy Sweet and Sour Cabbage (Tang Ts'u Pal Ts'*ai*)

2 lb.	*bok choi*
6	Chinese dried small red hot peppers
4 T.	cooking oil
2 t.	brown Sichuan peppercorns (*fagara*)
½ t.	salt
2 T.	brown sugar
3 T.	soy sauce
2 T.	brown vinegar
2 t.	sesame oil

Clean the cabbage and cut or tear into 2-inch squares. Cut the peppers in quarters lengthwise and discard the seeds. Heat the oil in a *wok* or skillet. Fry the pepper over high heat until dark brown. Add the brown peppercorns, stir for 1 minute, add cabbage, and cook for 3 minutes. When cabbage is cooked, add salt, sugar, and soy sauce. Stir. Add vinegar and sesame oil. Mix thoroughly and serve immediately or refrigerate and serve cold.

6 servings

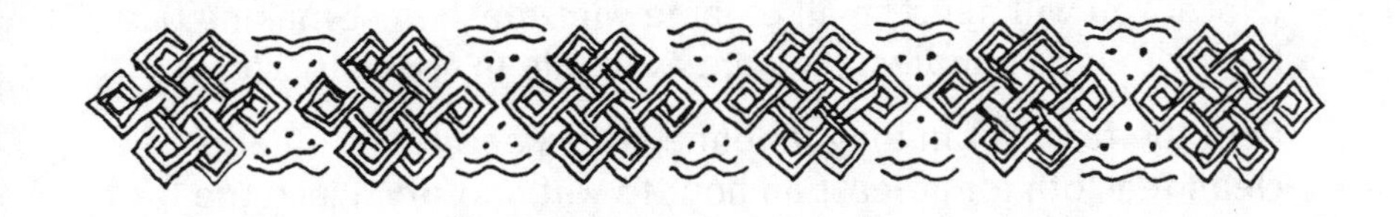

Stir-Fried Broccoli (Chao Chieh Cai)

2 lb.	broccoli
2 T.	peanut oil or safflower oil
½ t.	salt

1/2 t.	sugar
2 T.	water
1 t.	cornstarch dissolved in 1 T. cold water

Wash broccoli and separate the florets from stems. Discard the tough bottoms and peel the stems. Cut into 1-inch pieces. Heat the oil in a *wok* and add the broccoli stems. Stir for 1 minute and add the florets. Stir for 2 minutes, sprinkle with salt, sugar, and water, stir, and cover. Cook for 3 minutes. Uncover and add the cornstarch mixture until the broccoli is coated and shiny. Serve at once.

6 servings

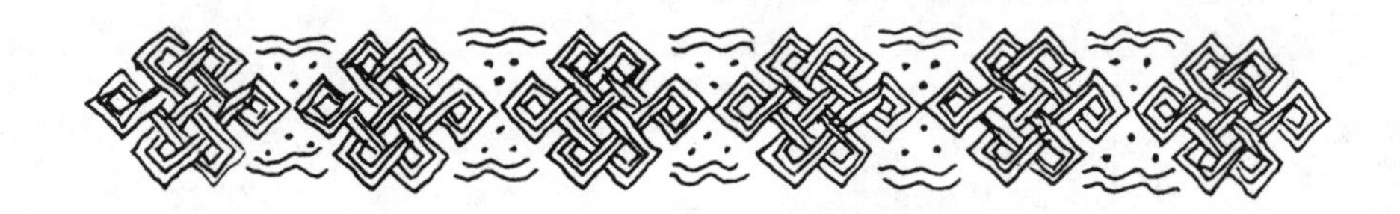

Taro Nests

1	large taro (3 inches to 4 inches in diameter, 8 inches to 12 inches long)
2 T.	soy sauce
1 T.	Shaoxing wine
2 T.	sesame seeds
	oil for deep frying

(Note: You will need small or large wire-mesh nest-making baskets with long handles; they are available in specialty stores.)

Peel the taro, cut in long julienne strips, and leave spread on a clean teacloth for at least an hour to wilt and dry. Place the taro in a large bowl and add the other ingredients to blend well. Heat the oil in a deep fryer. Twist the strands of taro together and place in slightly more than a single layer in the bottom of basket set. Cover with the insert basket and lower gently into the hot oil. Fry until lightly golden, then gently turn the basket over and remove, leaving the nest to brown uniformly. Remove the nest carefully and place on paper towels to drain and cool.

After the nests have air-dried and cooled they may be served filled or as an accompaniment or stored in an air-tight container for future use.

Large nests can be made by using 2 strainers as a form. This makes an attractive serving arrangement for any combination of stir-fried vegetables. *6–8 nests*

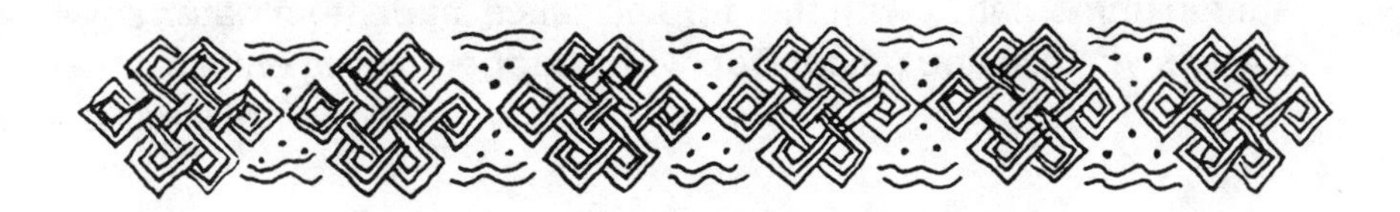

Steamed Vegetable Dumplings

3 C.	all-purpose flour
1 C.	boiling water (or substitute 36 prepared frozen steamed dumpling wrappers for first two ingredients)
3 T.	peanut or other oil
2 T.	sesame oil
1 1/2 C.	parboiled Chinese cabbage, chopped
3/4 C.	cooked bamboo shoots, chopped
3/4 C.	cooked water chestnuts, chopped
6	dried Chinese black mushrooms, soaked, rinsed, and chopped
1	cake firm-pressed white bean curd, cut salt and ground white pepper to taste

Dipping Sauce

1 T.	water
1 T.	soy sauce
1 T.	vinegar
1 T.	fresh ginger, minced chopped spring onions as garnish (optional)

Make a dough by mixing the flour and boiling water, then kneading it for 5 minutes when cool. Divide the dough into 36 pieces about the size of a tablespoon and roll into a thin circle. Place the oils in a *wok* and stir fry the cabbage, bamboo shoots, water chestnuts, and diced bean curd. Salt and pepper to taste. Remove the mixture from the *wok*, stir well, and place 1 tablespoon of the vegetable mixture in the center of each wrapper. Pinch the dough into a crescent shape. Arrange on lettuce leaves or cheesecloth in steamer and steam over high heat for 5 minutes. Serve immediately with the dipping sauce made from water, soy sauce, vinegar, and ginger. Top with chopped spring onions.

36 *small dumplings*

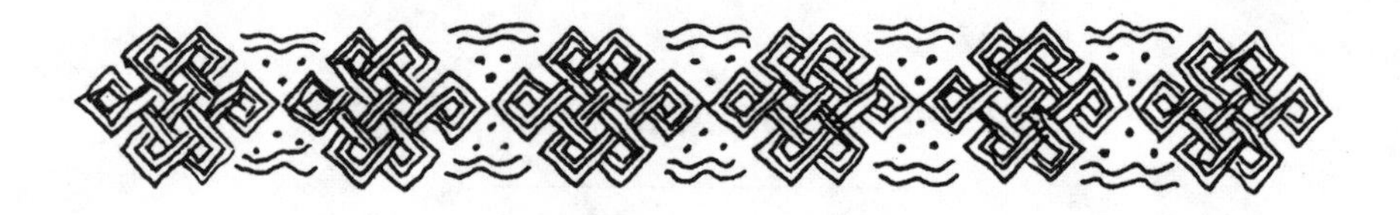

Stir-Fried Bean Curd and Vegetables

2	cakes pressed bean curd
2	carrots
4	stalks celery
1	sweet red pepper
2 C.	Chinese spinach, well rinsed
2 C.	soybean sprouts
6	spring onions
½ lb.	fresh mushrooms
4–6 T.	peanut or other cooking oil
	soy sauce, ginger, garlic, and sesame oil to taste

Cut all ingredients into matchstick strips. Heat the oil in a *wok* and stir fry all ingredients (except the soy sauce, ginger, garlic, and sesame oil) until desired doneness. Season with last four ingredients to taste and serve.

4 *servings*

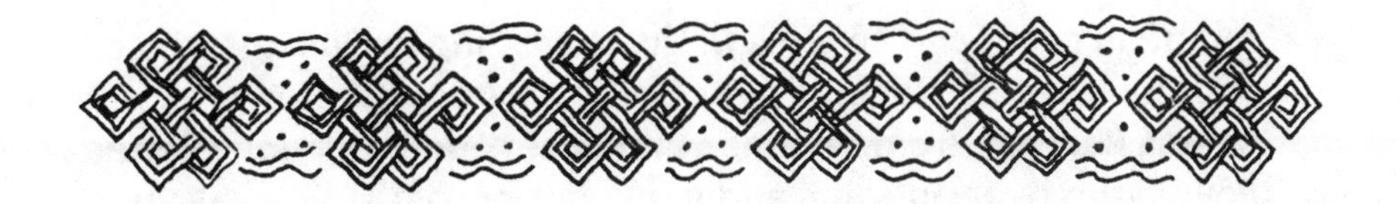

Eight Treasure Rice Pudding (Pa Bao Tian Fan)

Pudding

1½	C.	glutinous rice
2	T.	lard (margarine may be substituted)
2	T.	cooking oil (for greasing mold)
10		dried jujubes (Chinese red dates)
10		large pitted dates
20		candied lotus seeds
20		white raisins
20		almonds
¼	C.	candied orange peel, diced
¼	C.	candied citron, diced
¾	C.	red bean paste (canned)

Syrup

1	C.	water
¼	C.	sugar
1	T.	cornstarch dissolved in 3 T. cold water
1	t.	almond extract

Place rice in colander and rinse until water runs clear. Cook rice in 2¼ cups of water over high heat till it comes to a boil. Lower heat and cook until the water is absorbed, about 15 minutes. Add sugar and lard or margarine and mix well. Grease an 8-inch souffle or other heatproof dish. Take a few pieces of each of the following ingredients: dried jujubes, pitted dates, candied lotus seeds, white raisins, almonds, candied orange peel, and candied citron and place decoratively on the bottom of the heatproof pudding dish. Mix the remaining quantity into the rice. Place ½ the rice in the dish and flatten the surface. Spread with red bean paste and cover with the remaining rice mixture. Place dish in covered steamer over boiling water and steam for 1 ½ hours. Remove from steamer and invert onto serving platter. Pour syrup over pudding and serve hot or cold. To make syrup, boil 1 cup of water with ¼ cup sugar, 1 tablespoon cornstarch dissolved in 3 tablespoons cold water, and 1 teaspoon almond extract. Stir until smooth. *8 servings*

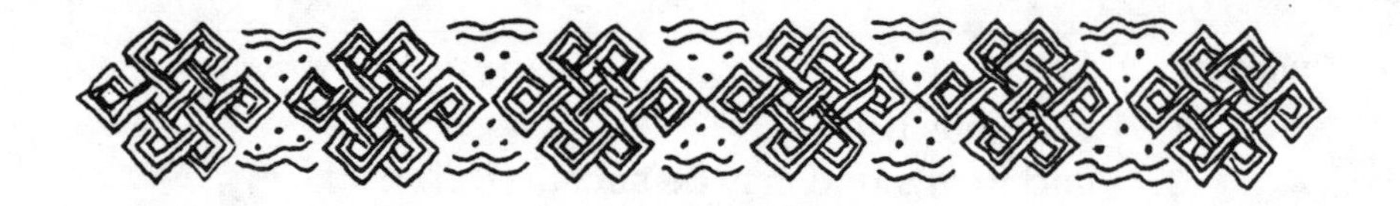

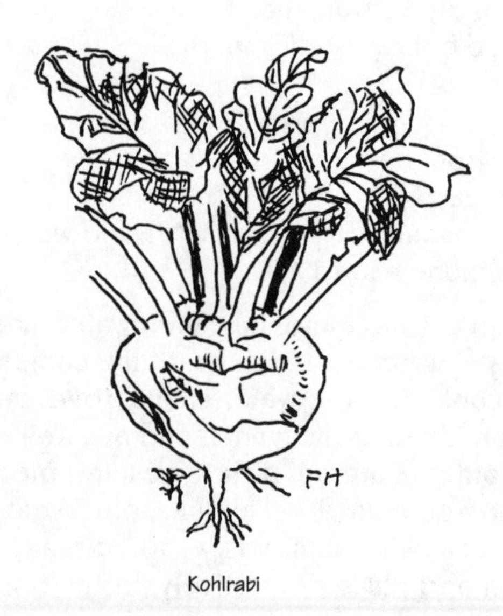

Kohlrabi

11

TEA AND YUM CHA

Among the plants and herbs the Emperor Shen Nung, the "divine farmer" (2737–2697 B.C.E.), named and described as beneficial was an evergreen, *camellia sinensis*. The tea lore tells that the emperor was meditating under the branches of a camellia tree and staring into the cauldron of water boiling over his campfire. The breeze brought camellia leaves down into the cauldron. The aroma enticed him to taste the brew and he found it enormously satisfying. *Camellia sinensis* grows wild in bushes fifteen to thirty feet high, with some reaching fifty feet. When they are cultivated, they are kept at heights of three to five feet. The white blossoms somewhat resemble the wild rose, and after the blossom drops, there is the tea fruit with three seeds.

Another story tells that the Bodhisattva Bodhidharma fell asleep while meditating. To prevent this from happening again, he cut off his eyelids (which seems a very un-Zen thing to do) and from them grew tea plants. From that time on, monks have drunk tea to stay awake.

Cha, the Chinese word for tea, originally meant any infusion; sailors picked up the southern regional version of *tsay*, which was altered to "tea." Tea was regarded a substitute for intoxicating drink, and the first teapots were modified wine jugs. In the Han Dynasty (202 B.C.–221 A.D.), tea was such a symbol of prosperity that ornate tea blocks were used as money.

Tea drinking reached its zenith in the T'ang Dynasty (618–907 C.E.) and was sometimes drunk with herbal additions, milk, and/or butter. It was believed that tea provided a person with physical energy, a calm mind, and clarity of attention when taken over a long period of time. Many people still find this to be true. Lu Yu wrote in *Ch'a Ching* (*The Tea Classic*) in 708 C.E.: "Tea tempers the spirits, calms and harmonizes the mind. Tea alerts thought and prevents drowsiness, lightens and refreshes the body, and clears the perceptive faculties."

In *The Chinese Art of Tea* John Blofeld says that Lu Yu referred to the apparatus used to collect spring water as a "well" and would never have used ordinary village well water, contaminated as it was with moss and other pollutants, to make tea. Mountain spring water was the best, then the water of the West River, and well water was a third choice.

In China, tea is presented with uncomplicated simplicity and in a relaxed atmosphere, almost a meditation on what the moment is. It is never empty ritual, but focuses on moments of goodness and consciousness.

In solitude or society, tea continues to be a medium for communication. In both domestic and social life, tea has the same importance in the most informal setting or in the most formal of state functions. Following is a list of typical Chinese teas.

Green Tea, Non-Fermented

Lee cha, or green tea, is the least processed of all teas; it is steamed until soft, then rolled and dried over charcoal. It does not ferment. It is best when steeped with water that has been just brought to simmer poured over it. It is brewed in two minutes, though with a fine-quality green tea one minute is perfect; a second brewing with the same leaves for a second cup will taste delicious, as the palate is already prepared for it.

Some Sichuan green teas, such as "green city," also known as "wife's father" (*chang jen*), and "hidden peak" (*meng ting*, the central peak of Mount Meng, clouded by the immortals to protect the delicate tea), are considered delicacies. "Cloud mist" grows high on the Kiangsi cliffs, and it is said that monkeys are trained to scale the perilous heights to bring the best leaves to the workers below. In the T'ang Dynasty in Chinkiang province, 30,000 young girls climbed the mountains before daybreak on early spring mornings to gather the leaves still covered in dew. In the valley, bells and cymbals were played to encourage them. "Dragon Well" (*lungjing*) is a popular, young green tea that has many beneficial attributes, as do the generic "gunpowder" teas available from contemporary packagers.

Green teas are delicate and should be purchased in small amounts as they do not store as well as more fermented teas. Storage is best in a tight-lidded caddy. The tea "caddy" is a name derived from *catty*, an approximation of a Chinese measure of weight that is the equivalent of 1.33 pounds.

Oolong, Semi-Fermented

Tung ting is mildly fermented oolong, almost like a green tea. "Iron goddess of mercy" (*Tea Kuan Yin*) will store for years. It is a Fukien tea, moderately fermented and grown near a temple dedicated to Kuan-yin. In the temple an iron statue of the goddess spoke to a local tea grower and told him the location of the finest tea shrub. It has kept the name.

"Iron Buddha tea" is from Chiuchow and is strong and bitter. It is considered good for the digestion and a benefit to health and strength.

Many famous oolongs came from Taiwan. In 1896, from what was then called Formosa, 20 million pounds of oolong were shipped to America under the name "Oriental Beauty." Oolong means "black dragon." It is said to be so named because children in the region where it is grown were frightened of the baby snakes that slithered on its shrubs. They were told by the adults that the snakes were baby dragons and the name stuck. It is a mildly fermented tea, as is the scented *pouching*, which is made with the addition of jasmine and gardenia blossoms.

There are also white oolong teas such as "white peony" (*pai mu tan*) and "noble beauty" (*ying mei*).

Flower Blends

Flower teas, such as *hua ch'a* or "scented slivers" and *hsiang p'ien*, are very popular. Since jasmine grows plentifully, it is the most popular flower for use in tea, with the chrysanthemum and the rose used with some frequency. In times gone by, gardenia, lotus, orchid, and plum blossom were used. Chrysanthemum tea is a cooling blood tonic in the summer heat and is regarded as a longevity tea. "China rose"—

black tea and rose petals—is considered a special-occasion tea. In Taiwan there is a green tea scented with chrysanthemum, as well as another with narcissus.

Black, Fully Fermented

Red teas, or *hung ch'a*, are what we call black teas in the West. The tea leaves are spread on a screen and dried by exposure to the heat of the sun or hot air. Then they are rolled to expose the juice and start the oxidation process. The leaves are left on cool surfaces made from glass, metal, stone, or tile and then heated over charcoal. They grow dark red as they ferment. These teas are also popular in the West, where milk and sugar are often added. By the late Ming Dynasty (1368–1644 C.E.) there was tea throughout Europe. These teas are strong enough to store under dry, dark conditions, and since they "travel well," they are a largely exported product.

Lapsang souchong is a strong, smoked black tea from Hunan. P'*u erh* teas refer to the teas of the Yunnan province and are the only group of teas not distinguished by color, but by region. They are regarded as having medicinal and nourishing properties that act as a digestive, expectorant, energizer, and life extender. It was the army of Kublai Khan that spread the benefit of these teas.

More recently, the National Cancer Institute released test results based on animal and population studies made in Shanghai that say green tea consumption reduces the occurrence of esophagal cancer. In Japan, studies showed a lower incidence of lung and stomach cancer as well as lowered blood pressure. One of the things the researchers found was that the polyphenol compounds in green tea lower cholesterol by stopping the production of enzymes that can produce carcinogens. Green tea contains the least caffeine of all the caffeinated teas, about half the amount of an equal volume of brewed coffee. It is also mildly anti-bacterial.

Tea is a more complex compound than had been thought. It contains twenty amino acids, twelve sugars, six organic acids, polyphenoic compounds, theophylline, some fluoride, vitamin C, and up to five percent caffeine.

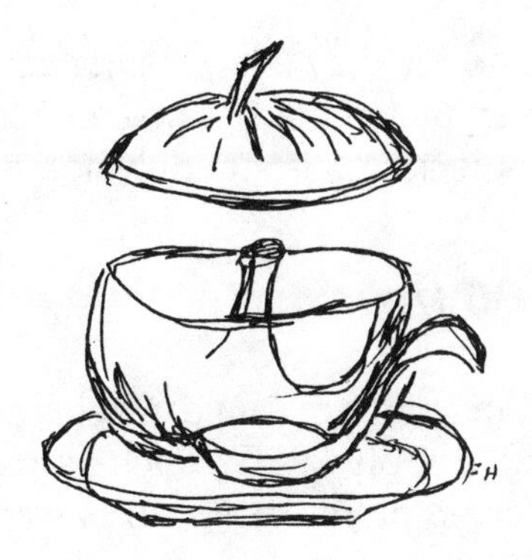

Individual Terra Cotta Steamers

'*Chung* are large cups with lids that are used either as a teacup or a vessel in which the tea is brewed and then drunk. The tea leaves settle to the bottom, and often the lid is slid to the side instead of being removed so that it holds back any loose leaves. In all parts of China today, people carry tea everywhere, in everything from thermos jugs to mayonnaise jars. On the street and in department stores, lobbies, train stations, and airports there are canteens of free hot water for making tea.

Lu Yu suggested that the best way to make tea is to boil spring water until you hear "the sound of majestic breakers." This water is to be poured over a quarter of an ounce of tea in a porcelain cup and then drained off. Add a second infusion of water, and that is the tea to drink. Some people still prepare tea this way. The modern way is to drink the first infusion.

In tea houses, the tea master will prepare special house blends that have gained a reputation, as well as traditional leaves. At home, approximately one ounce of tea to a cup of water steeped for three to five minutes will be the best way to test a new tea.

All the tea houses I have encountered, at every level of the economic scale, have been places of relaxed pleasure, and yes, the tradition of bringing caged birds to the shops in early morning still exists. Another less noticeable gesture is the tapping on the table with three fingers as an expression of gratitude to the pourer. This represents the time a Chi'ing Dynasty (1644–1911 C.E.) emperor himself poured tea when traveling incognito with his chancellors. To conceal his identity and yet acknowledge the honor they felt at being served by royalty, they made the gesture in emulation of the bowed head and arms in prostration. This sign of appreciation is still duly noted today.

Yum Cha

Dim sum is almost a sporting event in southern China, where there are hundred of combinations of items. Simple snacks such as peanuts, watermelon and lotus seeds, preserved plums, bean cakes, and dried fish are often served with tea. But it is *dim sum*, from the endless steamed and baked round buns we know in the West to wonderful surprises such as the soup-filled dumplings, that raises these snacks to an art form. *Har gau* is a good example, with the shrimp showing through the paper-thin translucency of a rice-flour wrapper. *Kuk*, or bean curd rolls, offer a great variety of tastes that emulate everything from duck to sausage. Another favorite, *woo kok*, or fried taro puffs, are like a round Chinese version of a French-fried potato. Everyone is intrigued by *ho yip fan*, the lotus leaf wrapped, tied, and filled with fried rice.

Some items are sweet, such as *nor mai chi*, or coconut cakes, and *dahn sarn*, or sweet, sticky cake with almonds. There is a version of thousand-layer cake called *chien chang go* that is very popular.

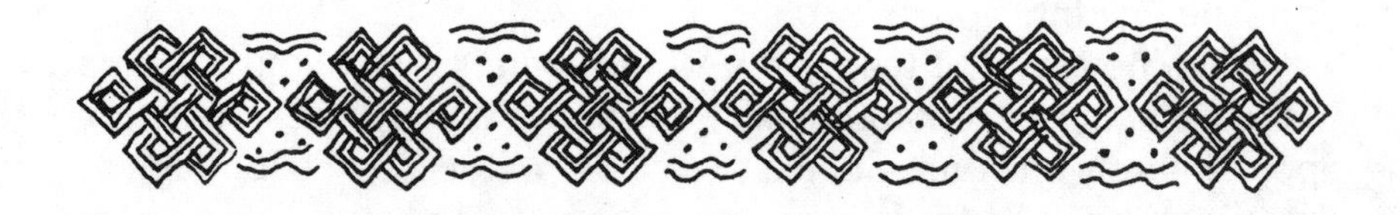

Fried Taro Puffs (Woo Kok)

2 C. taro (a little over a pound), peeled and diced
½ C. solid shortening
2 C. all-purpose flour (to be mixed with ½ cup boiling water)
1 T. sugar

1/2	t.	baking soda
1/2	t.	salt
1/2	t.	white pepper
1	T.	cooking oil
1/4	lb.	ground pork
1/4	C.	onion, diced
2	oz.	dried shrimp, soaked, drained, and diced
2	oz.	dried mushrooms, soaked, rinsed, drained, and diced
1/2	C.	water chestnuts (preferably fresh), diced
1/4	C.	water
2	T.	Shaoxing rice wine
		oil for deep-fat frying

In enough water to cover, boil the taro until tender. Drain, reserving 1/2 cup of the water, and mash the taro. Mix 1 cup of flour with 1/2 cup of boiling taro water. Blend with the mashed taro and add the other cup of flour and the sugar, baking soda, salt, and pepper till well blended. Set aside.

Place the cooking oil in a *wok* and saute the pork until cooked. Add the onion and saute, then stir in the shrimp, mushrooms, and water chestnuts. Blend in the water and wine. Remove from the *wok* and reserve until cool enough to handle.

Meanwhile, make golfball-sized portions of the taro dough. Place one portion in the palm of one hand and flatten slightly. Place one rounded tablespoon of the meat mixture in the center of the dough and re-form into a sealed ball. Repeat until all the dough and meat mixture have been used. Deep fry at 250° or, if using a deep fryer, follow the manufacturer's directions. Remove the puffs when golden brown, drain, and serve.

Yields 25 small puffs

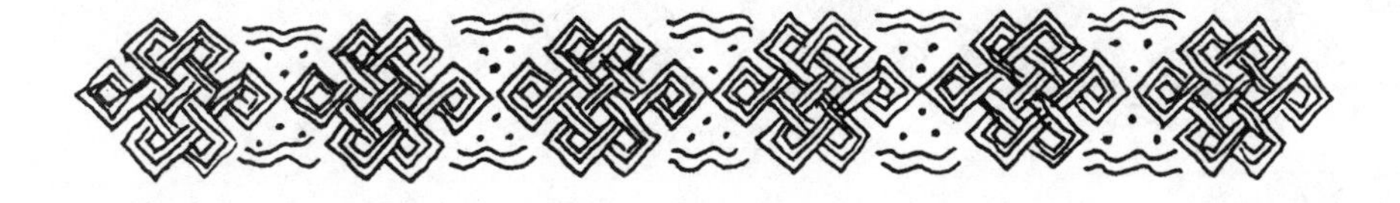

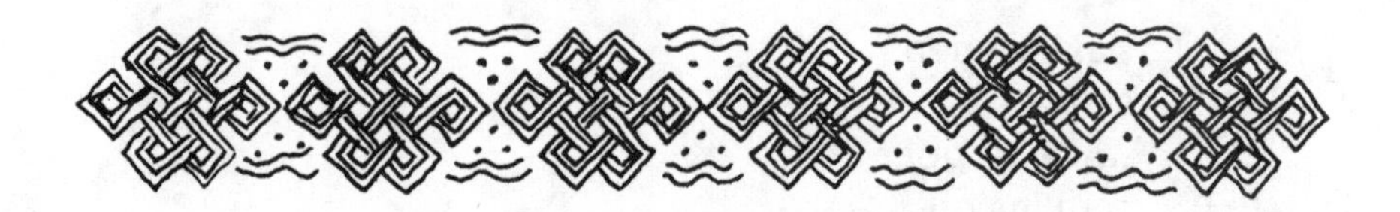

Bean Curd Rolls (*Kuk*)

2		cakes bean curd
1/2	C.	dried mushrooms, soaked, rinsed, and shredded
1/4	C.	carrots, shredded and parboiled
4		spring onions, shredded
1/2	C.	bean sprouts
1	T.	sesame oil
1	T.	sugar
		pinch of salt and white pepper
3		sheets of bean curd skins
2	t.	cornstarch mixed in 1 T. cold water
1	C.	cooking oil

Mash the bean curd cakes until smooth, and if there is any liquid, drain. Add the mushrooms, carrots, spring onions, and bean sprouts. Stir until blended, then mix in the sesame oil, sugar, salt, and pepper. Cut each bean curd sheet into four pieces. Divide the filling into 12 portions and place one on each bean curd skin. Fold into rectangles and seal with the cornstarch mixture. Place the cooking oil in a *wok* or skillet and fry the rectangles until crisp on each side. Drain on towel and cut each in half on an angle to serve. *Yields 12 rolls*

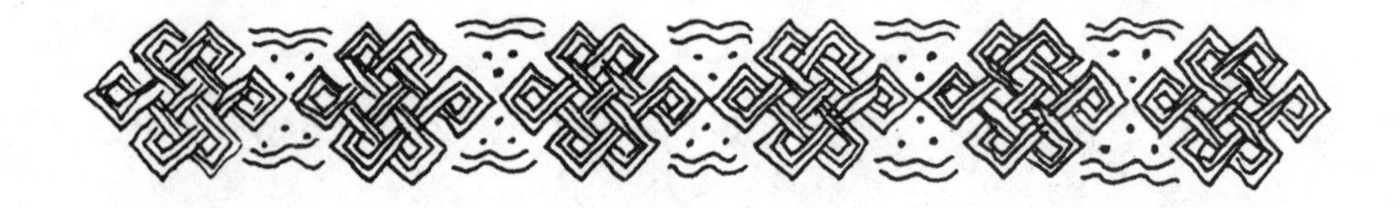

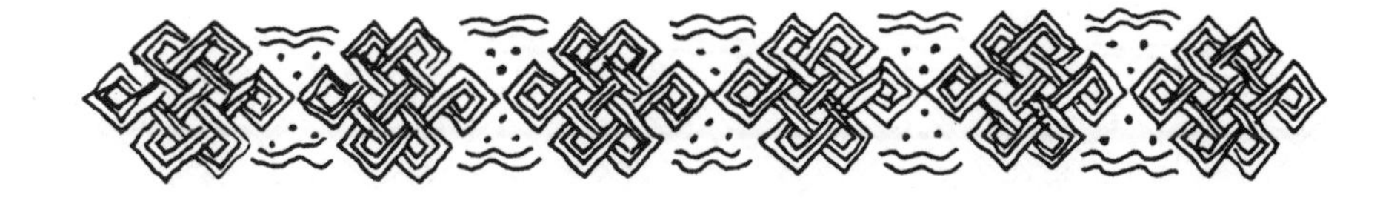

Steamed Shredded Buns

1	pkg.	dry yeast
1 1/4	C.	warm water
1	t.	sugar
3	C.	all-purpose flour
2	t.	baking powder
1/2	lb.	fat pork or slab bacon
1/2	C.	sugar
2	T.	ham, minced
2	T.	candied fruit, diced (optional)

Dissolve the yeast in the water with one teaspoon of sugar. Add to flour and knead until smooth. Cover and let rise 2–3 hours. After the dough has risen, add the baking powder and knead into the dough for 2 minutes. Roll the dough into a thin (about 1/4-inch) square about 24 inches on a side.

While the dough is rising, cut the pork or bacon into 1/2-inch pieces and cook until well done in a skillet or *wok*. Do not drain. Mix in the sugar and then spread the pork mixture on the dough sheet. Roll up jellyroll fashion. Put a steamer to boil. Cut the roll in shreds (about 1/3-inch slices). Take up six to eight shreds and form into a snail-shaped bun. Cover each bun with diced ham and fruit if desired. Place the buns on damp cheesecloth in the steamer and steam over high heat for 8 minutes. (These may be reheated the next day in a steamer for 3 minutes.) *Yields 12 rolls*

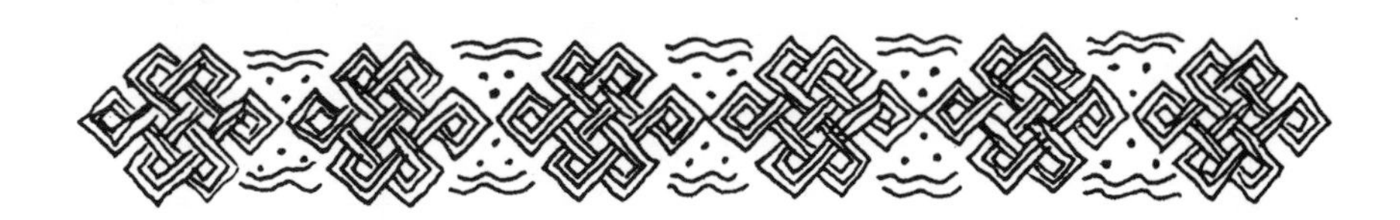

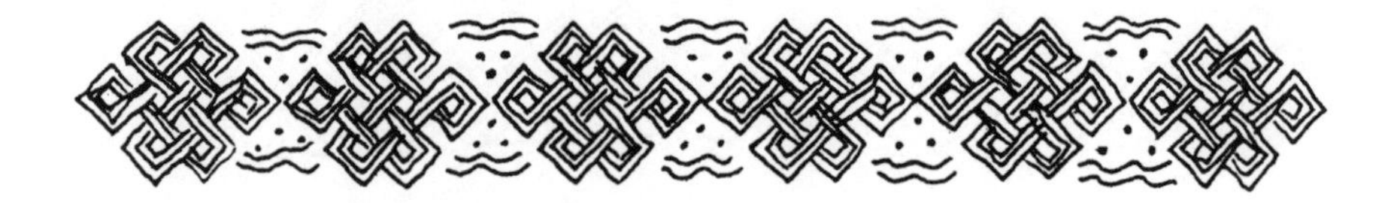

Spring Onion Pancakes

2	C.	all-purpose flour
1 1/2	C.	boiling water
2	T.	peanut oil
2	T.	sesame oil
1 1/2	C.	green onions, chopped
		salt to taste
1	C.	cooking oil

In a large mixing bowl, stir the water into the flour until it holds together in a rough ball. Knead for 5 minutes, adding the peanut oil toward the end of the kneading time. Cover the bowl with a damp cloth and let the dough rest for 1/2 hour. On a floured board, knead the dough briefly and form into 1 1/2-inch diameter log. Cut the log into about 12 slices 1 1/2-inch thick. Roll each slice into a 5-inch circle and brush the top with sesame oil. Sprinkle half of the pancakes with spring onions, salt to taste, and top with a second pancake, oiled side down. Press together with the oiled sides touching and then smooth with a rolling pin. Put a light layer of oil in a flat skillet on medium heat. Fry the pancakes 3 minutes on each side and serve hot. *Yields 6 pancakes*

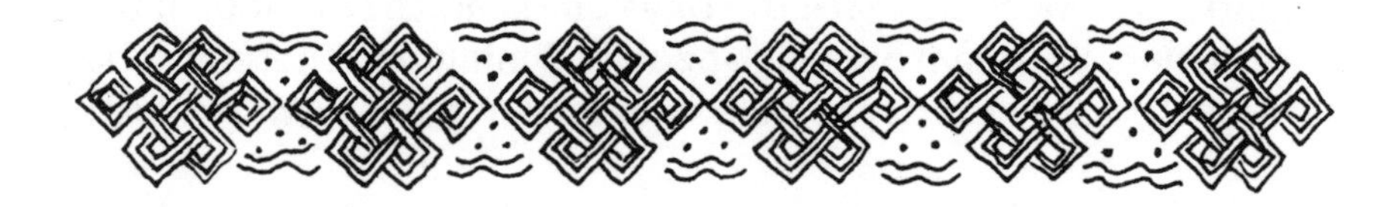

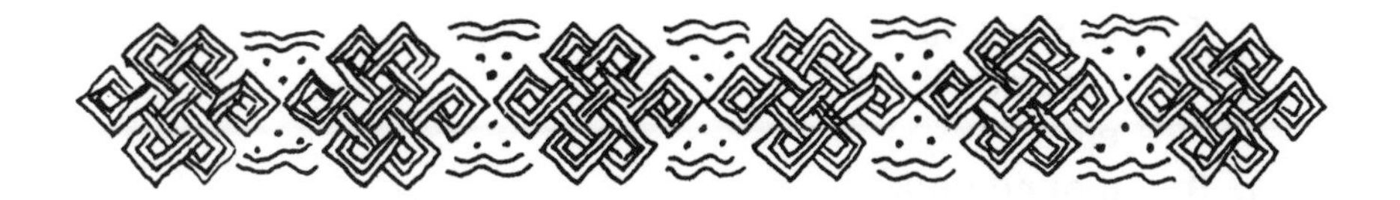

Turnip Cakes

2 C.	Chinese turnips, peeled and julienned
2 C.	rice flour
1 t.	salt
1/2 t.	white pepper
2 T.	sugar
1 1/2 C.	water
2	Chinese sausage, together about 1/4 lb., chopped

Boil the turnips for 5 minutes and drain. Place the rice flour, salt, pepper, and sugar in a cooking pot and stir in 1 1/2 cups of water. Mix until smooth, then add the drained turnips and the sausage. Place over medium heat on the top of the stove and bring to a boil, stirring constantly. Place the mixture in an oiled square pan and steam for 45 minutes. When the turnip cake is cool, slice and pan-fry. *8 servings*

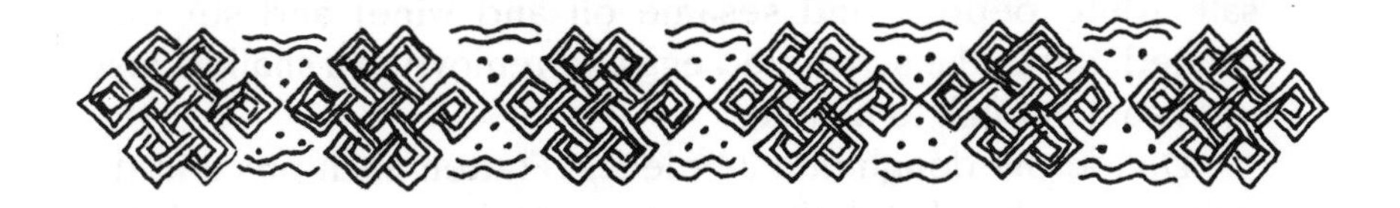

Fried Curry Rolls

1 pkg.	yeast
3/4 C.	warm water
2 T.	sugar
2 C.	all-purpose flour
1 T.	baking powder

1	T.	cooking oil
1	T.	sesame oil
2		eggs
½	lb.	ground pork
1	C.	onion, diced
½	C.	carrots, julienned
½	C.	spring onions, julienned
½	C.	dried mushrooms, soaked, rinsed, and minced
1	T.	plus 1 t. curry powder
1	t.	cumin
½	t.	salt
¼	t.	white pepper
2	T.	Shaoxing rice wine
1	T.	sesame oil
3	C.	fine bread crumbs
		oil for deep frying

Dissolve the yeast in the water and add the sugar. Place the flour in a bowl and pour the yeast mixture into it, mixing until smooth. Add the baking powder and oil and incorporate. Let the dough rest while the filling is prepared.

Heat the sesame oil in a *wok* and scramble the eggs. Remove the eggs and reserve. Stir fry the pork, onions, carrots, green onions, and mushrooms. Add seasonings (curry powder, cumin, salt, white pepper, and sesame oil and wine) and stir until cooked. Stir in the scrambled egg and remove to a shallow bowl until cool enough to handle.

Divide the dough into 24 pieces. Flatten each piece in the palm of one hand and place a heaping tablespoon of the filling in each one. Fold the dough to enclose the filling and pinch to seal. Place the bread crumbs on a shallow pan and roll the rolls in the crumbs. Heat the oil to 250° or, if using a deep fryer, according to the manufacturer's directions. Fry the rolls until they are deep golden brown, drain, and serve. *Yields 24 rolls*

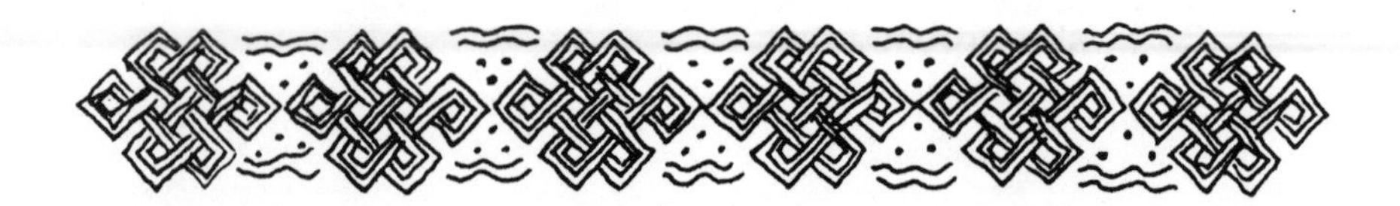

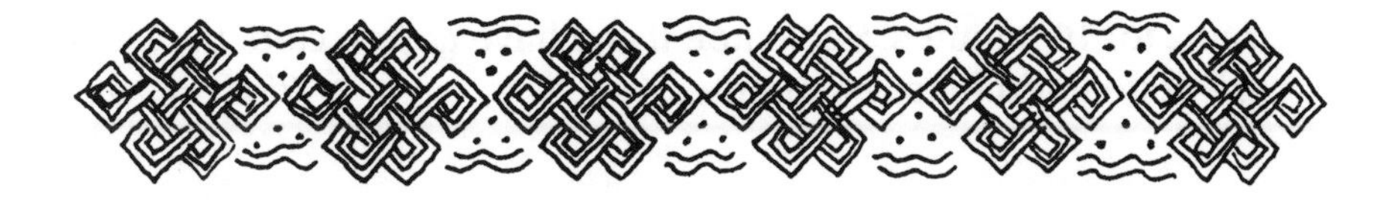

Steamed Roast Pork Buns (Ch'a Shao Pao)

1	pkg.	yeast
2	T.	sugar
1¼	C.	warm water
4	C.	cake flour
2	T.	cooking oil
1	T.	baking powder
¾	lb.	Chinese barbecue pork, julienned
1	t.	sugar
1	T.	soy sauce
1	T.	oyster sauce
1	t.	fresh ginger, minced
½	t.	star anise, ground
1	T.	plus 1 t. cornstarch dissolved in ¼ C. water

Mix the yeast, sugar, water, and 2 cups of the flour in a large bowl. Turn out onto a floured board and knead until smooth. Place the mixture back in the bowl and cover. Let it rise for 3 hours. Add the other 2 cups of flour, baking powder, and 1 tablespoon of cooking oil. Knead until well blended. Divide into 24 portions, and roll each into circles about 4 inches wide.

To make the filling, place 1 tablespoon of cooking oil in a *wok* or skillet and add the pork, sugar, soy and oyster sauces, ginger, and anise. When well mixed, add the cornstarch dissolved in water. Stir until the mixture thickens a bit. Then remove from the heat to a platter until cool enough to handle.

Place 2 tablespoons of filling on each dough circle. Pull the edges of the circle up to meet in the middle and twist slightly until the bun is closed. Set each bun on a square of parchment or waxed paper. Cover with a tea towel and let rise for a half an hour. After the buns have risen, set up a steamer and steam the buns for 10 minutes. Serve hot. If any have gotten cold, they can be resteamed for a few minutes. *Yields 24 buns*

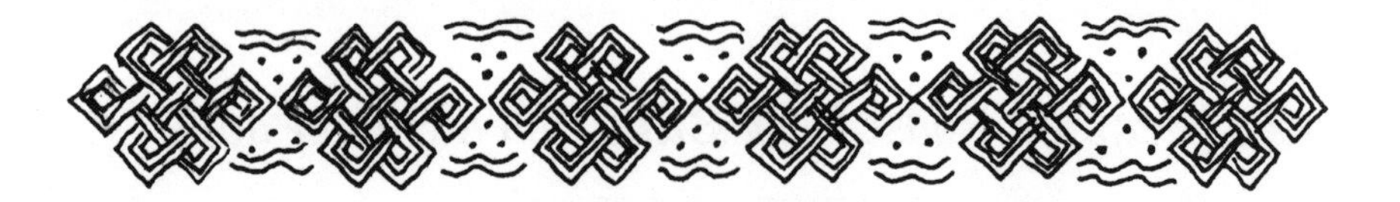

Baked Roast Pork Buns

Dough

- 2½ C. all-purpose flour
- ¾ C. water
- ⅓ C. lard or solid shortening
- 2 C. all-purpose flour
- ⅓ C. lard or solid shortening

Filling

- ¾ C. water
- 2 T. cornstarch dissolved in ¼ C. water
- 1 T. soy sauce
- 1 T. oyster sauce
- 1 t. sugar
- ½ lb. Chinese roast pork, diced
- 1 egg yolk

Preheat the oven to 375°. Mix 2½ cups flour, ¾ cup water, and ½ cup lard or solid shortening and knead for 3 minutes. This is the water-flour dough. Then mix 2 cups all-purpose flour and ⅓ cup lard or solid shortening and knead for 3 minutes. Divide each dough mixture into 24 pieces. Roll or press each water-flour dough piece into a 3-inch circle. Press a piece of the flour shortening mixture on top of it.

To make the filling bring the water to boil in a *wok* or saucepan and add the other ingredients. When slightly thickened, remove from the heat and cool enough to handle. Place the filling in the center of each combination dough circle and wrap. Pinch securely closed. Place the buns on a cookie sheet with the rounded side up. Brush with the slightly beaten egg yolk. Bake for 10–12 minutes, or until golden brown. Serve hot.

Yields 24 buns

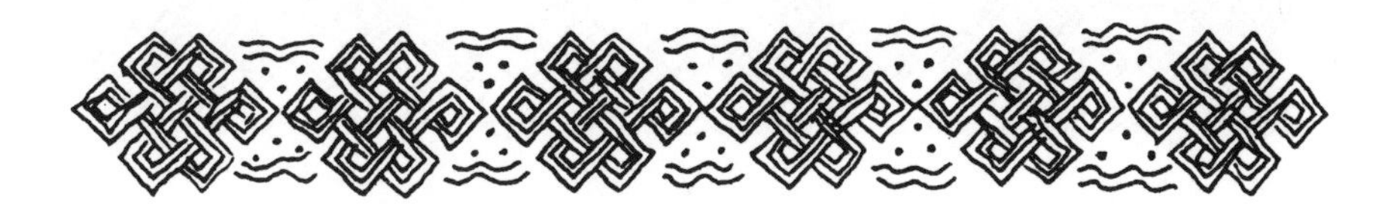

Vegetable Steamed Dumplings

Dough

(Prepared or frozen *wonton* skins may be substituted)

- 1¾ C. all-purpose flour
- 1 C. boiling water

Filling

- 1 C. *bok choi*, shredded
- ½ C. fresh-cooked bamboo shoots, diced small
- 3 T. dried black mushrooms, soaked, rinsed, and shredded.
- 2 T. cilantro leaves, minced
- 1 cake *dofu*, mashed

Place the flour in a mixing bowl and gradually incorporate the water. Cover it with a damp cloth and let rest for 30 minutes. On a floured work surface, knead the dough for 3–5 minutes. Divide the dough in half and roll into 2 logs, 1-inch across and 5-inches long. Slice each log into ½-inch pieces and roll each into a circle 3-inches to 3½-inches in diameter.

Set up a bamboo steamer and bring the water in the *wok* or base pot to boil. Mix the filling ingredients and divide into 20 portions. Place one portion on each circle, slightly stretch the dough around one half the circumference, and wrinkle slightly to meet the other half, forming small crescents. Practice is the only way to get this down. Place the dumplings in steamer racks, cover, and steam over boiling water for 10–12 minutes.

Yields 20 *dumplings*

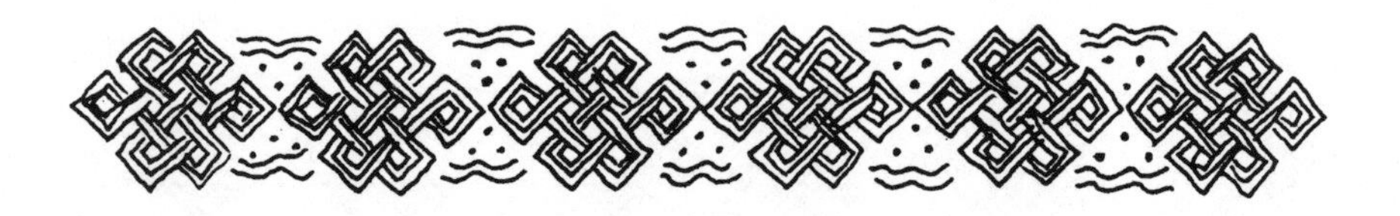

Pot Stickers

Dough

(Use dough recipe from Vegetable Steamed Dumplings)

Filling

1/2	lb.	ground pork
1/4	lb.	ground shrimp (pork may be substituted)
6		fresh water chestnuts, minced
1/4	C.	spring onions, minced
1	T.	soy sauce
2	T.	Shaoxing rice wine
1	T.	sesame oil
1	T.	fresh ginger root, minced
2	T.	parsley or cilantro leaves, minced
		salt and pepper to taste

Prepare the dough as in the recipe for Vegetable Steamed Dumplings. Mix the filling ingredients until very well amalgamated and divide among the wrappers. Seal in crimped crescents. Place in steamer racks over boiling water for 15 minutes. Remove and let cool. (They can be refrigerated till the next day.) Heat 3 tablespoons of peanut oil in a *wok* or skillet until sizzling. Place the dumplings in the *wok* and add another 3 tablespoons of peanut oil. Fry until the bottoms start to get brown and crisp. Sprinkle 2 tablespoons of water over all and cover to contain the steam. Reduce the heat and cook 4–5 minutes, checking once or twice to make sure the dumplings are not burning. Serve hot. *Yields 24 dumplings*

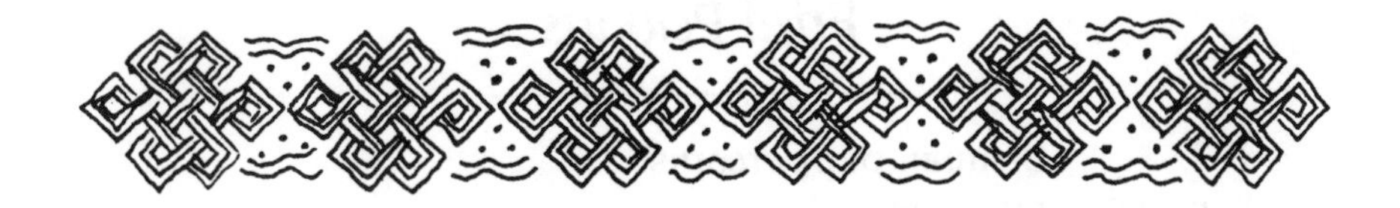

Marble Tea Eggs

8		jumbo eggs, hard boiled
3	C.	water
1	T.	black tea leaves
2	T.	soy sauce
1	t.	sugar
6	pieces	star anise
2	inch	cinnamon stick
1/2	t.	cracked peppercorns
3		strips mandarin peel

Holding each egg in the palm of one hand, tap it gently all over its surface with the back of the bowl of a wooden spoon until it has a network of cracks. Repeat with all the eggs. Make sure none of the egg shell is removed. In a non-reactive saucepan, place the remaining ingredients, bring to a boil, and lower the heat to simmer. Place the eggs in the mixture, cover the pan, and set on flame-tamer or other device to keep the heat as low as possible under the eggs. Cook for an hour. After an hour, remove from heat, leave the lid on, and let the eggs cool. Place them in the refrigerator for up to 24 hours. Remove the eggs from their shell before serving and cut into quarters or sixths.

Note: Variations of this recipe can be made with beets, oolong tea, or cinnamon as a colorant. Another possibility is green tea with lime peel and ginger. *Yields 8 eggs*

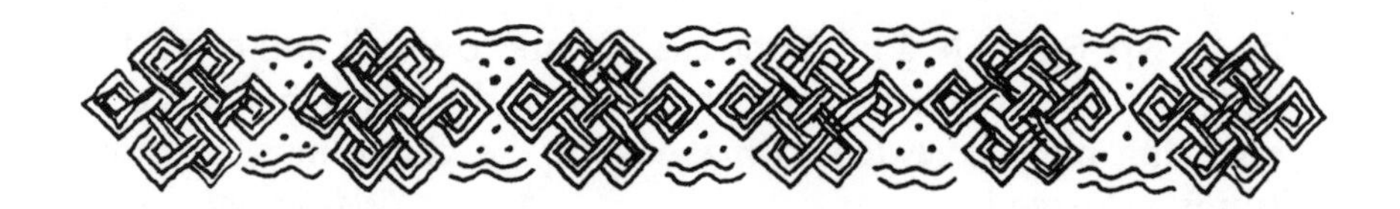

Fried Peanuts

1	T.	Sichuan peppercorns
8	pieces	star anise
1	t.	sugar
3	C.	water
2	C.	shelled raw peanuts
3	T.	sesame oil

Bring the spices to boil in the water. Add the peanuts, cover, and simmer for 5 minutes. Turn the heat off and let rest until cool. Place the mixture in the refrigerator for several hours or overnight. Drain the peanuts and pick out the pepper and anise. Rub the peanuts dry with paper towels. Heat the oven to 275°. Place the sesame oil on a cookie sheet and roll the peanuts in the oil. Roast for 7–10 minutes. Serve hot or cold.

Yields 2 cups

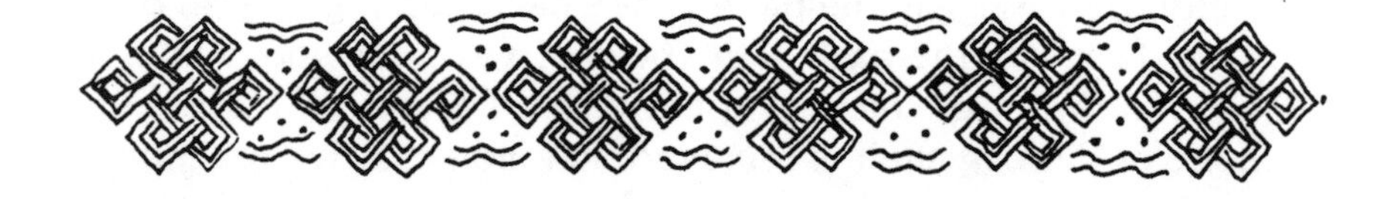

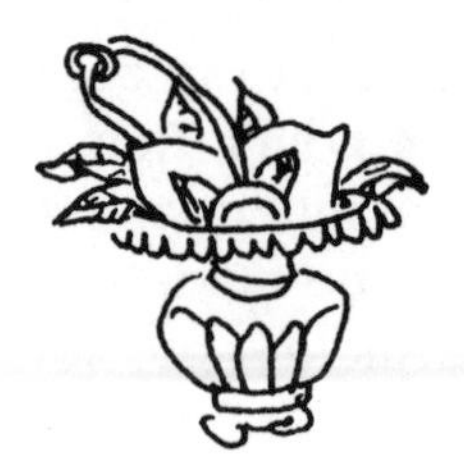

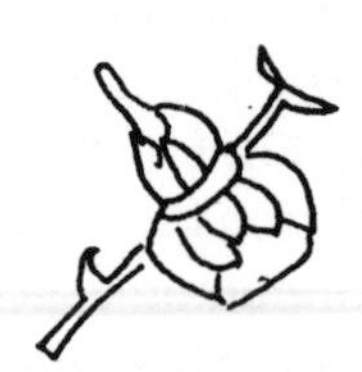

Taoist Symbols

12

Kitchen and Table

Cooking Tools and Techniques

In traditional Chinese kitchens there are usually square or rectangular tile counters into which are incorporated stoves with cook holes over which *woks* and pots fit. Some are like Indian *tandoori* ovens with the pots on top and the sides used for small breads. Many are like traditional European stoves and ovens that are a combination of wood and charcoal, and electricity, or gas. Some professional Chinese kitchens I have seen are so modern that they put many of ours to shame. A stainless-steel range top is available in the United States that has a built in *wok* well.

The basic cooking tools, though, have retained the same form as they have had for hundreds and, in some cases, thousands of years.

The Cleaver

Though I have been around professional kitchen equipment all my life, I haven't been so enthusiastic about a knife since I bought my first Sabatier in Paris. In Shanghai I bought one fine cleaver (*tou*) which is made of steel that holds a fine edge. It has an eight-and-one-half-inch blade (with the very barest curve) and is four inches at the handle and three and one-half inches at the tip. I chose one with a molded-steel handle that is of one piece, rather than one with a wooden handle. It handles like a fine etching tool, and I use it for everything but paring, boning, or slicing bread. I can't believe I managed without one. When you think that preparation is so important in Chinese food, it makes sense that the cooking tools are so satisfying.

As many dishes are meant to be cooked quickly, small uniform pieces are required. Slices, cubes, or matchstick strips are the most used. The cleaver will also mince, chop, pound and grind, blend, and pick up the food from the cutting board and let you slide it into the pot in one motion. Even when whole poultry, or fish, and large cuts of meat are cooked in one piece, cleaver cutting is required before serving. Knives at the table are considered vulgar. Keep your cleaver clean and dry.

Chopping Block

A chopping block is handy, although a good quality wooden cutting board will do. The traditional blocks are made from the cross-sections of soapwood tree trunks.

Special Cutters

Vegetable cutters with shaped blades for making intricate shapes are also useful for creating special effects. Dragons, phoenixes, leaves, fish, flowers, and geometric and calligraphic designs are cut into vegetables and melons and used to decorate baked dishes.

Wok

In Cantonese *wok* is simply the word for a cooking utensil. In Mandarin, it is *kuo*. It is designed with a full, round bottom because, for most of its 3,000-year culinary history, it fit snugly in the round opening of a wood or coal stove. With modern stoves, a collar or ring is used over the cooking hob to stabilize the *wok's* curved base. In China some chefs use a modified *wok* with a small, central flat base that contacts the heat source evenly. Usually these *woks* have a single handle, and they are a reasonable adaptation for modern cooking surfaces. Both versions are sold with covers, straining lips, and steamers to fit.

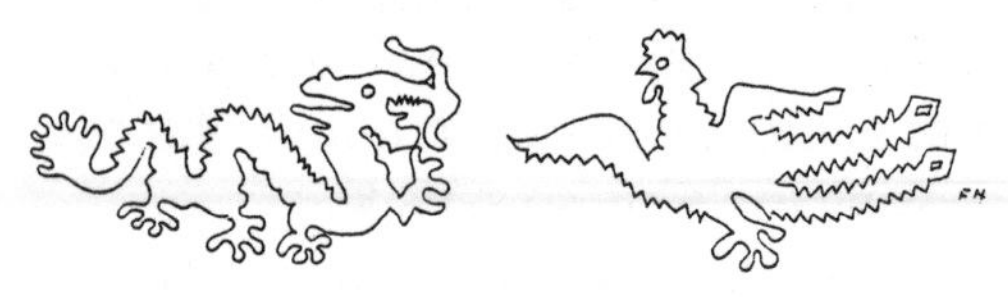

Dragon and Phoenix Vegetable Cutters

It is the cooking style that the *wok* makes possible that is important: a small amount of oil, small-cut ingredients, and a lot of motion—that's why they call it "stir fry." For use over electric hobs flat-bottomed *woks* are more dependable than the round-bottomed ones. The average cooking time for food in a *wok* is five to seven minutes. A minimal amount of hot oil sears all the ingredients, and then a bit of liquid, stock, sauce, or water completes the cooking.

Long Chop Sticks

These are used to place food in the *wok* and stir it as it cooks. They are also used to place food from the *wok* on a serving dish.

Wok Sang

This is a shovel-like spatula that is used because it can manipulate large amounts of food in the *wok* to insure even cooking.

Brass Strainers

Various sizes of wooden-handled, flat-disc-shaped strainers are helpful. They will lift and drain the food from oil or water and are large enough to hold the food while you add something else to the pot.

To practice using a *wok*, add two tablespoons of cooking oil to a *wok* (prepared according to the manufacturer's directions) over high

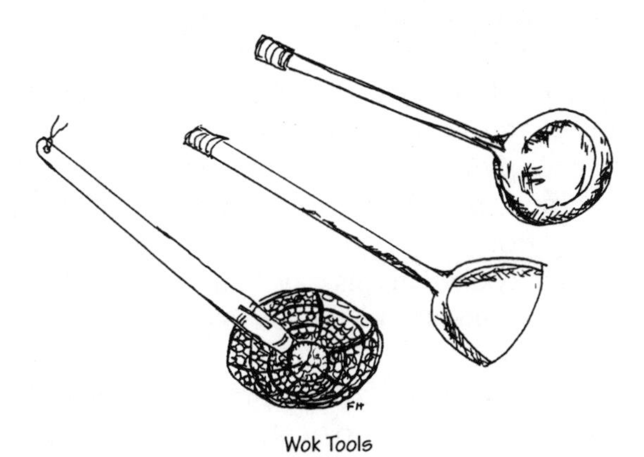

Wok Tools

heat. Wait until the oil is just starting to sizzle, about a minute or two. Spread the oil over the *wok* by tilting it or with the *wok sang*. This way, no food will touch any raw metal and burn. Do not lift the *wok* to distribute the oil, as this will cool it. Add the vegetables and stir them with the *wok sang* until they are coated. You will see the vegetables change color as they cook. Add some flavoring and liquid that will steam the food a bit. Cover the *wok* for about three minutes. Uncover and test the vegetables for desired doneness. If you want to add a special sauce or wine, this is the time to do it. Stir it to blend and serve immediately.

This is the principle of most Cantonese *wok* cooking. In the North and Sichuan, the process is similar, but often the cover is not used.

Red Cooking

One of the combination methods used with a *wok*. Large cuts of poultry, fish, or meat can be browned in a small amount of oil. They are then removed and placed in boiling water for a while, taken from the water with a skimmer, and returned to the *wok* with a brown sauce, then covered and braised.

Most common cooking methods can be accomplished with a *wok* and a cleaver. With the addition of various components, they are used to stir-fry, deep-fry, pan-fry (sauté), simmer, boil, or steam. They can even be used to roast.

Steamer (Ching Lung)

Steamers usually fit over *woks* and the rising steam heat cooks the food. Often they are made of bamboo and can be stacked four high, although rarely more than that. They can be used with lettuce leaves or cheesecloth squares covering the bottom of each section, leaving a rim of open space. Some food can also be prepared, cut, and marinated or sauced and, on a heat-proof plate, put in the steamer directly. Everything from meat, poultry, and vegetables to *dim sum*, bread, and buns are cooked in this way. You can also fit steamers over a stock pot, leaving your *wok* free, or you can use a modern stainless-steel stacked steamer.

Chinese stewing is similar to steaming. In a pot with a tight-fitting lid, the ingredients for a soup or stew are placed as to be cooked

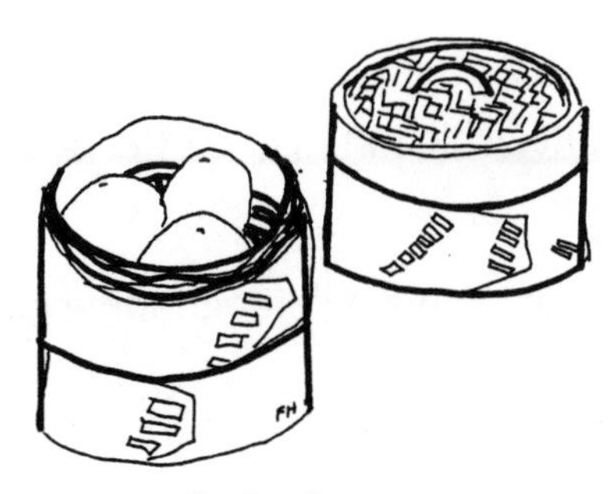

Bamboo Steamer

over a flame. Instead, the pot is placed in a larger pot with water up three-quarters of the sides. Both pots are covered and the water is brought to a boil. Then the heat is lowered and the food is cooked over medium heat until done.

A steamer can be improvised by placing two or three heat-proof cups or a flat-bottomed bowl upside down in a stock pot with boiling water on the bottom and setting the dish to be steamed on top. The pot is then covered and the food is steamed until it is cooked.

Sand Pots

These are casserole dishes, usually with one handle, that are unglazed on the outside. They are very good for stews and thick noodle dishes and are meant to be used on top of the stove. Most of the food is cooked first, added to the pot, seasoned, and set over heat to become fully cooked and blended.

Mongolian Hot Pot

This has a central chimney holding charcoal that boils the water in the pan set around it. Each diner selects finely sliced food from a platter and holds it in the water with chopsticks until it is cooked, much like *fondue*. Condiments and accompaniments are placed on the table, and the food is seasoned to taste. At the end, soup is made from the resulting broth by adding vegetables. This is then served in individual bowls.

Miscellaneous

Chinese rice paddle, which will get all the rice from the pot to the serving plate
Large soup ladle
Mortar and pestle or simple mill for grinding grain or spices
Paring knife
Small rolling pin

One of the things that an early exposure to Chinese cuisine taught me is that the simpler and fewer my tools were, the more I could pay attention to cooking. If the ingredients are on hand, a large meal can be easily prepared in less than an hour. Some devices are as handy as a *sous chef* and, in addition to the items mentioned above, a food processor, a pasta machine, an electric deep fryer, and a rice cooker might assist the home cook in large-scale preparation. I also use, on rare occasions, an open electric grill with a rotisserie attachment that does not offer the aroma of open-fire grilling, but will serve nicely for some kinds of barbecue.

The Table and Tradition

For eight to ten people (and more), a meal might start with four to eight cold dishes. On a formal occasion, tea and small tidbits, such as sweet-and-savory nuts and seeds, are served before the cold course. Then follow four to eight hot dishes, accompanied by rice and/or noodles. After that comes soup, a savory and/or a sweet, and then fruit and possibly eight-treasure pudding or another similar dish. The food is served on platters, and in public circumstances, each platter has its own serving utensils, as food sanitation is respected and understood.

Informally though, people will use their chopsticks to help themselves from a platter. The etiquette involved is as it would be anywhere: you take the morsel you touch. There is no poking around and with dexterity, your chopsticks never touch anything but the food you are taking.

From plain platters of freshly cooked dishes to elaborate food sculptures, the presentation is never ignored, and as a matter of fact, it is literally the centerpiece of the meal. The visual (*se*, or color) and aromatic (*xiang*) components are regarded to be as important as taste

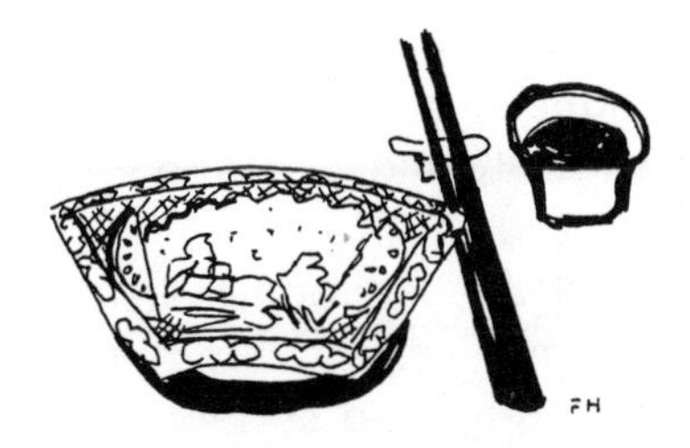

Individual Place Setting

(*wei*) to the pleasure of eating, along with good conversation and good humor.

At each place at the table there is a set of chopsticks. They are made most often of bamboo or plastic, but you can also find them in lacquered wood, jade, ivory, and even silver and gold. As in the West, when the host or hostess raises their chopsticks, it is time to begin. When the meal is finished, the chopsticks are left across the rice bowl. Even slightly formal tables are round and seat from eight to twelve people. If there is a single host, he or she usually sits facing the door with the guest of honor, if there is one, on the right. The second host sits opposite, with the second guest of honor on his or her right. Otherwise, if there are two special guests, they sit on either side of the host. The rest of the seating is dictated by any logic one wishes to use. Sometimes the host starts by serving some food to the people on either side as a token, just to get the ball rolling. But even in restaurants where there is a high degree of service, it is traditional to help yourself from platters and bowls, often placed on a central lazy susan. There is a sociability about this common usage that prevents dining experiences from becoming stiff.

If liquor is served, it is usually the host who begins the toasts, saying "*gan bei*," or "dry cup," the Chinese equivalent of "cheers." It is not polite to drink alone, but if you do not want to drink, it is perfectly fine to raise your glass or cup in a return gesture but not actually drink. You can do the same when you want a drink, offering the toast and then drinking after the gesture has been returned. There is more of a fixed tradition to this than with food formalities. Meals in China tend to be relaxed and conversational, and tea service is casual, even when the setting is elegant. Banquets can be ritualistic and filled with subtle flattery and snubs based on rank and importance. At most family and holiday banquets, wherever they are held, the air is easy, the hosts and guests circulate and chat, and everyone is made to feel "at home."

In addition to chopsticks, a spoon is usually provided at each place setting. The traditional ceramic flat-bottomed spoon is being replaced by a metal round-bowled spoon. There are rests that are specifically designed to hold chopsticks and spoon that are very decorative. They are often in whimsical animal shapes, such as elegant lions or fish. Cloth napkins are now used almost everywhere, and many street restaurants offer paper napkins. In many restaurants and in some private homes, hot cloths are passed once or more during the meal to refresh hands and mouth.

Though platters and serving bowls can be very large, individual plates are usually no more than ten inches in diameter. An open bowl about ten inches in width is also used for noodles or *congee*, but not soup. Soup is served in a bowl only a little larger than a teacup. The rice bowl is a little larger than the soup bowl, but of the same shape. The smallest cup is used for wine. Of course, this may vary, but is generally the case. There are also assorted condiment dishes and cruets, as well as teapots, wine jugs, and the inevitable toothpick holder. Toothpicks are considered proper at the table. Polite form is one hand wielding the toothpick in subtle motion, with the other hand held as a veil in front of the mouth.

Standard tableware can certainly be used, but the Chinese service adds another dimension of pleasure as well as practicality. Soup, for

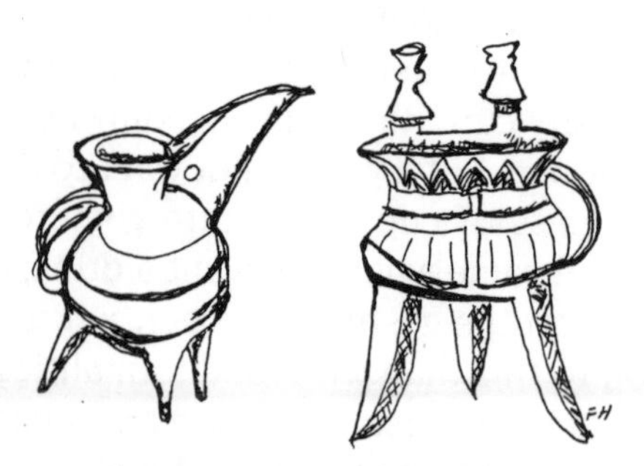

Antique Water Jar and Wine Jug

instance, gets cold and gelatinous in shallow Western soup plates. In the deep Chinese bowls, especially when covered, the soup stays hot and the texture remains satisfying. Yuan Mei (1715–1797) has been called the Brillat Savarin of China and he offers the following good advice.

> Don't make your thick sauces greasy or your clear ones tasteless. Those who want grease can eat fat pork, while a drink of water is better than tasteless soup. Don't over-salt your soups, because salt can be added to taste, but can never be taken away.
>
> Don't eat with your ears; by which I mean do not aim at extraordinary out-of-the-way foods, just to astonish your guests. That is to eat with your ears, not with your mouth. *Dofu*, if good, is nicer than bird's nest. Better than sea slugs which are not first rate is a dish of fresh bamboo shoots.
>
> The chicken, the pig, the fish, and the duck are the four heroes of the table. Sea slugs and bird's nests have no characteristic flavors of their own, but are usurpers in the house. I once dined with a friend who gave us bird's nests in bowls more like vats, each holding about four ounces of the plain boiled article. The other guests applauded but I smiled and said, "I came here to eat bird's nest, not to take delivery of it wholesale."
>
> Don't eat with your eyes. By which I mean do not cover the table with innumerable dishes and multiply courses indefinitely. This is to eat with the eyes and not with the mouth.
>
> A good cook cannot turn out more than five distinct dishes. I used to dine with a friend who served twenty-four dishes and sixteen sweets. My host delighted in this, but when I got home I was so hungry I used to have a bowl of *congee*.

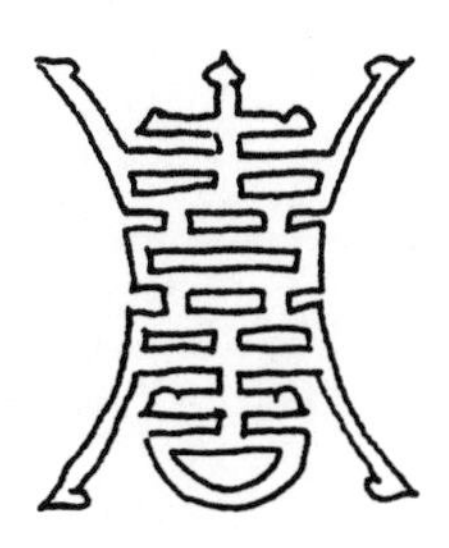

Symbol for Happiness

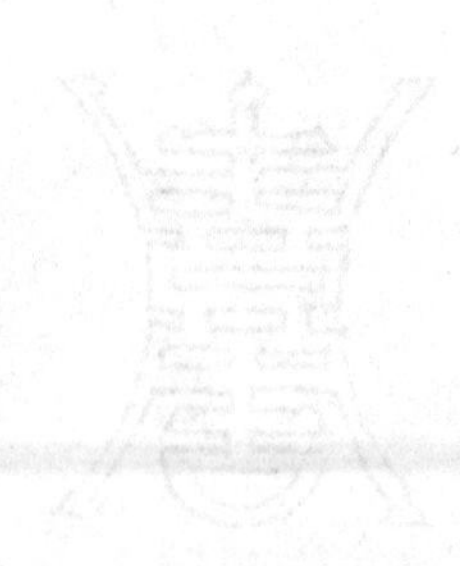

13

INGREDIENTS

Abalone (canned): Once opened, rinse and use immediately. They are best in sauteed dishes.

Abalone (dried): These store well. Soaked and then sliced or minced, they are used in soups or clay-pot dishes.

Agar agar: This is a natural gelatin made from seaweed; usually used to make desserts.

Bamboo shoots: All bamboos produce shoots, but only one out of ten species are good for eating. Bamboo shoots can be bought prepared at many Chinese specialty stores. Otherwise, peel them and discard the heavy root base. Boil the shoots for twenty minutes. They should be tender and have no bitter taste. If they taste tough and/or bitter, slice them and cook again for another 5 minutes. Use the shoots immediately or store in the refrigerator in frequently changed water for up to two weeks.

Bean curd (dried): White or brown (from five-flavor seasoning), these can be cubed or shredded and used for dishes such as Sichuan noodles. They are good in stir fries and soups as well. Refrigerate them well wrapped in plastic film.

Bean curd (fermented): This is very pungent and has been likened to aged cheese. It is usually sold in jars and used as a condiment. It will keep, covered in its brine, for several months in the refrigerator.

Bean curd (fresh): Processed soybeans are pressed into custard-textured squares of about three inches. They can be kept in water in the refrigerator for two weeks if the water is changed daily. This is the base for *mapo dofu* and other high-protein dishes.

Bean curd skin (dried): These are stiff sheets of bean curd that keep well out of the refrigerator. They are soaked and used as wrappers for various fillings.

Bean sprouts: Fresh mung bean sprouts are about one-and-one-half inches long. The fresh are best by far and should have no brown spots. To use, remove the parchment husk and any minute green leaves and prepare immediately. They may be refrigerated in a covered container in water that is changed every couple of days for up to two weeks. The canned ones should be used only when necessary and not kept more than a day or so after opening.

Bird's nest (dried): Usually sold in small packages or by the pound, these are used as a base for soups or one or two desserts. They keep almost indefinitely in a clean, dry, air-tight container.

Black beans: Fermented, black beans are sometimes preserved with the addition of garlic and ginger. A small amount will season vegetables or fish. The beans in packaged plastic are better than the canned ones. Once the package is opened, the beans will store well in a covered container in the refrigerator. Before using, it is best to rinse them first (to remove excessive salt) and then to crush or chop them slightly. It is best to buy the ones without other ingredients because it is easy and more flavorful to crush them with some garlic, chili pepper, a touch of soy sauce, and sugar to get an instant black-bean sauce.

Black mushrooms (dried): As large as one or two inches across, these mushrooms do not resemble the European dried mushrooms. They keep well. Soak clean, drain, and then slice or mince.

Brown bean sauce: This sauce is made of whole or ground yellow soybeans, flour, water, and salt. It is slightly pungent and is used as a thickener for sauces or marinades. Remove it from the can and store in a well-washed and rinsed jar with a tight cover.

Chili paste: This is made from very strong ground chili peppers and salt. It is often packaged premixed with other ingredients such as garlic or fermented black beans, so read the label. It is always hot. It will keep in the refrigerator indefinitely.

Chili peppers: Generally speaking, the smaller the pepper and the smaller its "shoulder," the hotter it is. However there are certainly hot, round green peppers, and it is better to inquire or test timidly any pepper you don't know. Dried peppers can be stored for up to a year (some say longer) in an air-tight container. The fresh ones should be used within a couple of weeks. They can, of course, be used to make aromatic oils and other condiments, as well as cooked directly with food. To cook, heat several dried peppers in one cup of peanut or safflower oil to 375°. Keep at that temperature for about five minutes, being careful not to burn the peppers. Cool and store.

Chinese parsley: Also called coriander or cilantro, this herb is more aromatic than parsley. It can be stored standing in a tall glass with water in the bottom to cover the roots. Another way is to wrap the roots in a damp paper towel, tie it, and place in an inflated plastic bag. This herb is high in vitamins and minerals when fresh. It is best discarded when wilted or even a little brown.

Cinnamon: Chinese cinnamon is sold in large, slightly curved pieces that are milder in taste and aroma than the tightly curved variety we are accustomed to seeing in the U.S. Large pieces can be used in sauces and condiments and should be removed before eating. They are also used this way in braised and roasted dishes. The pieces can be ground and used as a flavoring for many dishes. Cinnamon is also an ingredient in the traditional five-spice mixture.

Conpoy: These are dried scallops. They keep well. To use, they are soaked and sliced thin. They are often used with fresh scallops in sauteed dishes.

Five-fragrance powder: Star anise, clove, fennel seed, cinnamon, and Sichuan peppercorns (*fagara*) are used in this seasoning. It is used especially in marinades for beef that is to be served cold.

Five-spice powder: This is a ground mixture of star anise, fennel seed, clove, Chinese cinnamon, and Sichuan pepper. It is sold in jars or can be made from scratch.

Fungi: Varieties of edible Chinese fungi grow on trees. "Cloud ear fungus," which has no stem, is the smallest. Wood or tree ears are thicker and a bit larger. They are sold dried in packages or by the pound and must be soaked and trimmed before using. They are prepared and used like mushrooms and stored the same way. They add a distinct woodsy overtone and texture to many dishes.

Garlic: Look for firm, unblemished heads. They are best stored with air ventilation in a cool place. The Chinese method of peeling garlic is similar to the French. The broadside of the cleaver is smashed down on the cloves, and they are slipped from their husks. I have not found any prepared garlic in oil preparations that I like. I have, on occasion, heated a bland oil such as safflower and added to it as many parboiled and carefully dried and peeled garlic cloves that it will cover. When the oil is cool, I put it in a covered jar and refrigerate it.

Ginger: It is best when bought relatively fresh with a paper-thin skin that is pale tan or golden in color. One-half inch to one inch is the best size. If a whole "hand" is bought, it will keep, although it will dry if kept for a few weeks. For use, peel, shred, slice, or mince. It can also be pressed for its juice. To store, peeled, cut ginger will keep well stored in Shaoxing wine for a couple of months in the refrigerator. I have found minced ginger will freeze in baggies, and though it is not as good as fresh, it is better than powdered or none at all.

Hoisin sauce: This is made from sugar, vinegar, soybeans, flour, water, salt, and a chili-spice blend, as well as sometimes from ground

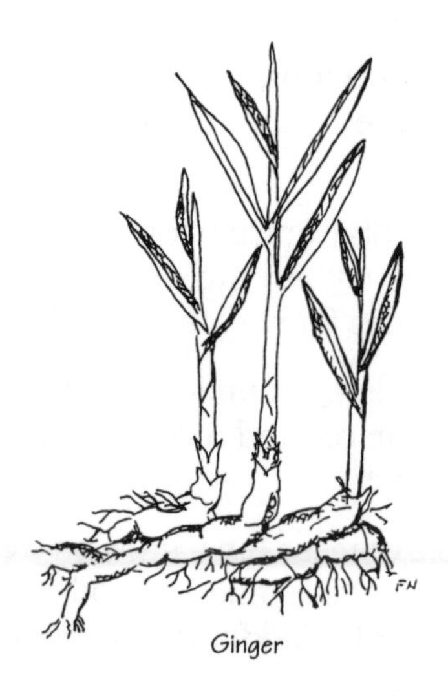

Ginger

sesame seeds, red beans, or garlic. Store it in a covered container in the refrigerator after opening. It will keep for a couple of months. This sauce is used a lot in Cantonese cooking to thicken and season food. Try to find brands without msg.

Jellyfish: This is sold either dried or packed moist and salted, shredded or in flat discs. They have a nice texture for salads and noodle dishes.

Jujubes: These are small, dried red dates sold by the box or pound. They have a unique flavor and are used in many Chinese sweets. They are usually an ingredient in any eight-treasure combination.

Kao liang: Sorghum made into mash then distilled.

Lily stems: Sometimes called the golden needle vegetable, they are tiger-lily buds. They keep almost indefinitely. Soak fifteen minutes and drain before using.

Lotus leaf: The dried sheets are sold in packages. These leaves are used to wrap steamed dishes and glutinous rice dumplings. They are soaked for an hour and then used whole or cut into the desired shape. They are not eaten.

Lotus root: This can be found fresh, dried, canned, or candied. Fresh lotus root will keep two weeks in a perforated plastic vegetable bag. The canned ones are poor substitutes and should be used within twenty-four hours of opening.

Mandarin zest (dried): Made from the dried peel of small oranges or tangerines, this is used in savory dishes to add a sweet, tart taste. It should be soaked for fifteen minutes before using.

Noodles: Egg noodles can be bought fresh at some Chinese specialty shops and will keep several months in the freezer. Others are sold dried by the pound or in packages. There are also frozen ones. They are cut from the very fine "dragon's whiskers" to broader varieties. Store the same way you do any pasta. Rice stick noodles (brittle noodles made from white rice flour), yellow wheat flour noodles (fresh or dried), cellophane noodles (made from mung beans), spring roll wrappers, *wonton* wrappers.

Pickles: There are various jars of pickles in any Chinese specialty store. Often they are preserved vegetables, such as mustard greens.

These are usually packed with chili, salt, and spices and should be rinsed before use. Various cabbages and green beans are also pickled. There are also sweet pickles such as ginger and watermelon rinds that can be eaten as an accompaniment. They are modestly priced, and you can try different ones until you find a kind you like.

Plum sauce: This is a preserve-like, plum-based sweet-and-sour sauce that is sold in jars or cans. It will keep on shelf until opened, then should be refrigerated.

Red rice: This is a form of wild rice.

Rice (long-grain): *Indica* tends to be light and fluffy when cooked or steamed. Uncooked rice will store in an air-tight container almost indefinitely. For three cups of rice, rinse one cup of long-grain rice, drain, and place in a two-quart pot with two cups of water. Bring to a boil. Boil for two to three minutes, cover the pan tightly, lower the heat, and simmer for fifteen minutes. Remove from the heat and let stand still and covered for ten minutes more. If you are using an electric rice cooker, follow the manufacturer's directions.

Rice (short-grain): Glutinous or sweet *Japonica* rice is stickier and starchier than long-grain rice and is used more frequently in Japan. It becomes very sticky and opaque when cooked. Glutinous rice is used for *sushi*, stuffing, and desserts.

Sea cucumber: These are dried sea slugs that are sold by the pound. They keep well dry, but must be soaked for at least twenty-four hours before using.

Sesame paste: Ground sesame seeds made in an aromatic oil that is different from the Middle-Eastern variety.

Sesame seed oil: Use the aromatic Chinese oil only. The Western or Middle-Eastern varieties may not be substituted. The darker it is, the thicker and stronger the taste. There is a debate over whether or not it should be refrigerated. I think a good idea is to store a large bottle in the refrigerator and decant a small amount a few hours before using it.

Sesame seeds: Miniscule, flat, oval shiny seeds. They are sold by weight, either black or white. They are often roasted either in a *wok* or oven to bring out their aroma.

Hot sesame oil: This is also aromatic sesame seed oil but with chili peppers or chili extract blended in. Use sparingly, as it can be quite hot.

Shaoxing (rice wine): This wine comes from Zhejiang province and is aged three to five years. When it is cooked, the alcohol evaporates and leaves a fragrance that enhances and blends the other flavors of a dish. It is never meant to be overpowering. It is the wine of choice for most cooked dishes requiring wine. Do not substitute Japanese wines, but dry sherry is acceptable. It will keep unopened almost indefinitely, and refrigerated open bottles will keep for at least a year if they do not evaporate.

Shark's fin: There are no substitutes for the dried shark-fin cartilage that is sold in dried strips or small triangles. It will keep dry indefinitely.

Shrimp (dried): These very tiny dried shrimp are used to flavor both sauces and fillings in rice and noodle dishes. They vary in intensity and price, and it is best to taste one before buying. I have successfully substituted tiny Alaskan shrimp sauteed dry and then seasoned with oyster, fish, or anchovy sauce.

Sichuan pepper: *Fagara*, as it is commonly called, is a mild pepper with aromatic overtones. It is best roasted slightly and freshly ground, or when ground and mixed with coarse salt to become a dip or seasoning salt.

Sichuan red-bean paste: This is salty and spicy, not sweet. Remove it from the can and store in a well-washed and rinsed jar with a tight cover. It will keep for several months. It is used to thicken and flavor dishes.

Sichuan red-bean paste (with chili peppers): This is the same as above, but with chili peppers added.

Soy sauce: Most soy sauce is made from fermented soybeans, wheat, yeast, sugar, and salt. The two standard ones are dark and light. The dark sauce is more syrupy and is used in braising and basting. The light sauce is sometimes used to thin the dark sauce. Light soy sauce is used for sauces and dips. In China it is not used much straight from the bottle as a condiment for rice, as it is in the United States or in

Japan. There are also blended soy sauces, such as mushroom, shrimp, or anchovy. By and large, these sauces only seem saltier. Do not substitute Japanese soy sauce.

Star anise: An eight-pointed star when whole, each point of the plant's star is a pod for a tiny seed. Used whole or ground, it is similar to fennel seed.

Sugar: Amber-colored Chinese sugar usually comes in blocks. It is a little less sweet than standard granulated sugar. It will keep in a tightly covered jar; if necessary, it can be softened in a microwave if it gets too hard to separate. I divide it into small portions, wrap each in plastic film packets, and keep the packets in an air-tight container.

Sugar (malt): This sugar comes in a crock and can be used like honey.

Sweet red-bean paste: This paste is made of red beans, sugar, and some shortening. Transfer it from the can to a clean covered jar in the refrigerator, where it will keep for a few weeks. It is used as a sweet filling for buns or other desserts.

Vinegar: Zhejian (Chinkiang) vinegar from Kiangsu province has the richest flavor. It is similar in its way to balsamic vinegars and can be used as a base for hot or cold sauces.

Vinegar (white): Made from rice, this is similar to Japanese rice vinegar. It is mild and used for cooking.

Water chestnuts: A little larger than a ping-pong ball, these are usually seen in Chinese markets coated with the soil in which they grew, much the way potatoes used to be sold. They can be stored as they are and cleaned before use. Or, they can be scrubbed, peeled, and stored in salted or sugared water, covered in the refrigerator until ready to use. Canned water chestnuts are as poor a substitute as canned potatoes are for fresh. Water-chestnut flour is used as a thickener for soups and stews.

GLOSSARY

By and large, *pinyin* is the English alphabet-based system of transcribing Chinese words so that they can be sounded out. The following chart indicates the way the letters are pronounced using international phonetic symbols.

A Comparative Chart of the International Phonetic Alphabet and the Chinese *Pinyin* Alphabet

b	[p]	z	[ts]	ia	[ia]
p	[p']	c	[ts']	ie	[iϵ]
m	[m]	s	[s]	iao	[iau]
f	[f]	a	[A]	iou	[iou]
v	[v]	o	[o]	ian	[iϵν]
d	[t]	e	[γ]	in	[in]
t	[t']	ê	[ϵ]	iang	[iaη]
n	[n]	i	[i]	ing	[iη]
l	[l]	-i (前)	[λ]	ua	[uA]
g	[k]	c (后)	[ʃ]	uo	[uo]
k	[k']	u	[u]	uai	[uai]
(ng)	[η]	ü	[y]	uei	[uei]
h	[x]	er	[ər]	uan	[uan]
j	[tç]	ai	[ai]	uen	[uϵn]
q	[tç']	ei	[ei]	uang	[uaη]
		ao	[au]	ueng	[uəη]
x	[ç]	ou	[ou]	ong	[uη]
zh	[tʂ]	an	[an]	üe	[yϵ]
ch	[tʂ']	en	[en]	üan	[yϵn]
sh	[ʂ]	ang	[aη]	ün	[yn]
r	[ʐ]	eng	[əη]	iong	[yη]

Useful mealtime words and phrases

"*Ni Shir-le fan le mai-yo?*" "Have you eaten yet?" used the same as: "Hi, how are you?"

"*Huan ying.*" "Welcome."

"*Xie Xie.*" "Thank you."

"*Qing.*" "Please."

fanguar restaurant

fanting dining room

chufang kitchen

luguan hotel

chifan to eat a meal

zaofan breakfast

wufan lunch

wanfan dinner

chi to eat

hé to drink

chizi spoon

chazi fork

daozi knife

kuaizi chopsticks

panzi plate

diezi saucer

fan a meal

é hungry

"*Wo é le.*" "I am hungry."

ke thirsty

"*Wo ke le.*" "I am thirsty."

"*Goule.*" "Enough."

shiyong de edible

gei to give

gei qian to pay

gui expensive

caidan menu

"*Wo keyi yao yi ge caidan ma?*" "May I have a menu?"

nashoucai specialties

"*Jintian you shenme cai?*" "What dishes do you have today?"

"Qing ni jieshao jiyang nimende hao cai ba." "Please recommend some good dishes."
"Nimen yo may yo . . . ?" "Do you have . . .?"
"Qing ni gei wo . . ." "Please bring me . . ."
"Gei wo. . ." "I want . . ."
duo yi dian . . . more . . .
shao yi dian . . . less . . .
kuai yi dian fast(er)
man yi dian slow(er)
"Hen hao chi." "Tastes very good."
"Ren ching wei." "The flavor of human feeling."
"Hao ji le." "Very good."
"Feichang bu hao chi." "Terrible food."
mama huhu so-so (literally horse, horse tiger, tiger)
yi diandian a little bit
duo yi dian more
"Deng yi deng." "Wait a moment."
"Gan bei!" "Cheers!" (literally dry cup)
youyi friendship

Yum cha Tea and snacks

cha tea
he cha to drink tea
lu cha green tea
moli ua cha jasmine tea
wu long cha oolong tea
ju hua cha chrysanthemum tea
re shen cha ginseng tea
cha bei teacup
wan cup with no handle
chaju teaset
chaguan teahouse
chadian light meal
yum cha tea and snacks (literally to eat tea)
jiaozi dumplings
hundun *wonton*

chun juanr spring rolls
da mi zhou rice *congee*
cai shao bao steamed bun filled with barbecued pork
chang fen savory stuffed fried sticky rice flour buns
jian dui zai sweet fried balls of rice flour stuffed with red bean paste
lo po gao fried turnip cakes
yu jiao fried savory stuffed mashed taro balls
luo mi ji lotus leaf wrapped glutinous rice, usually filled with chicken and dried shrimp and mushrooms
zongzi glutinous rice wrapped in bamboo leaves
cha ji dan tea eggs
shi zi tou "lion's head" meatballs, usually pork, shrimp, and ginger
dim sum (Cantonese) dot the heart
tien hsin touch the heart
yuebing mooncake (various: lotus, nut paste, candied fruit, bean paste fillings)
you tiao twisted cruller, "oil stick"
shao bing flat baked wheat bun, usually with sesame seeds
tian dianlei sweet snack (dessert)

Some basic ingredients

dan egg
dou bean
ya duck
e goose
gui yu salmon
qui yu Mandarin fish
li yu carp
yu fish
yu chi shark fin
yan wo bird's nest
ji chicken
huo ji turkey
xia shrimp
pang xie crab
long xia lobster

xiaoyang lamb
gaoyang mutton

Mian fan lei Rice and noodles

mi fan plain white rice
chao fan fried rice

Noodles are cut into sizes that vary from the very fine "Dragon's whiskers" to one inch broad flat noodles.

mi fen rice stick noodles, (white rice flour brittle noodles)
mian yellow wheat flour noodles (sometimes, egg noodles) fresh
gan mian yellow noodles, dried
si fen cellophane noodles, made from mung beans
chao mian fried noodles

Dou fu lei Tofu (bean curd)

dou fu bean curd
dou fu gan dried bean curd
fu yu fermented bean curd
hong shao dou fu braised bean curd
ma po dou fu Sichuan style
xing ren doufu sweetened bean curd with almond flavor

Jianguo Nuts

ru shu gao cashews
hua sheng peanuts
song zi pine nuts
hutao walnuts

Qing cai lei Vegetables

shu cai vegetables
bai cai cabbage

qin cai celery
bo cai spinach
shui qin watercress
dong gua winter melon
qing dou green beans
cong green onions
dou ya bean sprouts
zhu sun bamboo shoots
bi qi water chestnuts
shi zi jao sweet pepper
qie zi eggplant
xi hong shi tomatoes
yu mi xu corn
jiaomu yeast
cong spring onions
da suan garlic
qing cong shallots
tung kua chung winter melon pond, soup cooked in melon
yan sui cilantro (fresh coriander also known as Chinese parsley)
dai suen leek
choeng spring onion (also known as scallion or green onion)
mo gu mushroom
yin er cloud ear fungus
mu ehr wood ear fungus

Flavorings and sauces

yan salt
huhiao pepper
you oil
xiang you sesame oil
jiang ginger
wu xiang ten five-spice powder
tang cu zhi sweet-and-sour sauce
tian mian jiang *hoisin* sauce
mu li jiang oyster sauce
jiang you soy sauce

mei zi jiang plum sauce
pao cai pickles (general)
xiao hui xiang fennel seeds
la-jiao chilies
gui pi cinnamon
ding xiang cloves
xiang cai coriander
cu vinegar
tang sugar

Cooking methods

tang lei soup
lengpan cold dish
tan huo kao barbecue
zhu boil
bao ch'ao stir fry
kao roast
pao very fast frying
tan shu de poach
men long slow cooking
tun cooked as though in the top of a double boiler
zheng steaming
liji boneless

Shuiguo Fruit

guozi fruit
ping-guon apple
xing zi apricots
ju zi orange
li zi plum
xiang jiao banana
jin ju kumquats
tao zi peach
you zi pomelo

bo luo pineapple
li zhi lichee
mang guo mango
wuhuag guo figs
ying tao cherries
zao zi date
ning meng lemon
pin tao grape
shi zi persimmon
shi liu pomegranate
li pear

Yinliao Beverages

yi ping kuangquanshui a bottle of mineral water
kuang shui mineral water
qi shui carbonated water
ning meng qi shui lemonade
ju zi zhi orange juice
bing cha iced tea
pijiu beer
jiu wine
hong putaojiu red grape wine
bai putaojiu white grape wine
Shaoxing rice wine
bai lan di brandy

DIRECTORY

Airlines

China Airlines
630 Fifth Avenue
NYC NY 10111
PHONE: 212 399 7877

Cathay Pacific - Dragon Air
590 Fifth Avenue
NYC NY 10011
PHONE: 212 819 0750

Air China
45 East 49 Street
New York NY 10017
PHONE: 212 371 9898

ITT *Sheraton* Hotels

Worldwide reservations in the
United States and Canada
Toll free Phone: 800 325 3535

Great Wall Sheraton Hotel Beijing
North Donghuan Road, Beijing
PHONE: 86-1-500-5566
FAX: 86-1-500-1938

Sheraton Xi'an Hotel
12 Feng Gao Road, X'ian
PHONE: 86-29-426-1888
FAX: 86-29-426-2188

Sheraton Hua Ting Hotel
1200 Cao Xi Bei Lu, Shanghai
PHONE: 86-21-439-1000
FAX: 86-21-255-0830

Sheraton Guilin Hotel
Bing Jiang Nan Road, Guilin
PHONE: 86-773-282-5588
FAX: 86-773-282 5598-308

Lai Lai Sheraton
12 Chung Hsiao East Road, Taipei
Section 1
PHONE: 886-2-321-5511
FAX: 886-2-394-4240

Sheraton Hong Kong Hotel &
Towers
20 Nathan Road, Kowloon
PHONE: 852-369-1111
FAX: 852-739-0521

Restaurants

Beijing

Li Family Restaurant
(reservations only)
11 Yang Fang Hutong
Denei Dajie, Xi Cheng, Beijing
People's Republic of China

Joy Guest Restaurant (see text for directions)
Beijing, People's Republic of China

Yuen Tai Restaurant
Great Wall Sheraton Hotel
North Donghuan Road
Beijing 100026, People's Republic of China

Fangshan Restaurant
Beihai Park
Beijing, People's Republic of China

Shanghai

Guan Yue Tai Restaurant
Sheraton Hua Ting Hotel

Huxinting Teahouse
in Yu Yuan Garden

Shanghai Lao fandian
(Old Shanghai restaurant)
242 Fuyou Lu (near gate of Yu Yuan Garden)

Gongdelin Vegetarian Restaurant
43 Huanghe Lu

Meixin Resturant
314 Shaanxi Nanlu

Xinya Restaurant
719 Nanjing Donglu

Meilongzhen Sichuan Restaurant
1081 Nanjing Xilu

Guilin

Guilin Food Street *Du Xiu Cun* and Chinese Restaurant *Guo Tai*
Sheraton Guilin Hotel

Friendship Dining Hall
Zhongshan Zhonglu

Yueya Restaurant
located in Qixing (seven star) Park

Ying Shi Liu Dong Miao (Buddhist Temple)
Li Sa Chan Ting, the Buddhist restaurant located in Xishan Hu Park

Xi'an

Tang Student Institute, decorated and costumed in the period
Qu Jiang Chun
192 Jiefang Lu

Defachang JiuJia (dumpling) Restaurant
Dong Dajie, Pingan Market (near the Bell Tower)

Wuyi Fandian
351 Dong Dajie

Gongdelin Vegetarian Restaurant
Miaohou Jie

Dao Xue Mian
Tumen Dajie

Qingyazhai Restaurant (*paomo*)
Dong Dajie

Taipei

Happy Garden Restaurant
Lai Lai Sheraton
12 Chung Hsiao East Road,
Section 1
Taipei, Taiwan

Tien Hsiang Lo Restaurant
The Ritz Hotel
41, Min Chuan E. Road, Section 2
Taipei, Taiwan

Fu Yuan Restaurant
No. 17 Lin Ye Street
Taipei, Taiwan

Din Tai Fung
194 HSIN-1 Road, Section 2
Taipei, Taiwan

Chyuan Sheeng Vegetarian
Restaurant
111 Linsen N. Road
Taipei, Taiwan

Hong Kong

Celestial Court Restaurant
Sheraton Hong Kong Hotel and
Towers
20 Nathan Road, Kowloon, Hong
Kong

Snow Garden Restaurant
233 Electric Road,
Northpoint, Hong Kong

Cleveland Szechuan Restaurant
6 Cleveland Street
Causeway Bay

Golden Island
25 Carnavon Street
Tsimshatsui, Kowloon

Sun Tung Lok Shark's Fin
25 Canton Road
Tsimshatsui

Tsimshatsui *night market* (after 7
p.m.)
Haiphong Road *daipaidong* street
food stalls; after 8 p.m. food
stalls, shopping, and street
entertainment

Yua Ma Tei night market
Temple Street *daipaidong* street
food stalls, shopping, and street
entertainment

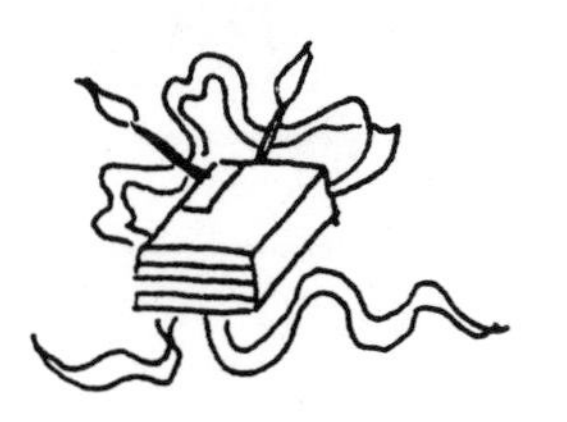

Art Symbols

General Index

Recipe Index

Beef

Buns, Dumplings, and Pancakes

Chicken

Congee

Desserts and Sweets

Duck

Fish